The Law of Rhythmic Breath

(1908)

Teaching the Generation, Conservation, & Control of Vital Force

Partial Contents: Breath is Life; Master-key of creation; How to gain & use the master key; Evolution of the Tattvas; Happiness vibrations; Manifestations of Prana; Planetary influences upon the Tattvas; Activities of the macrocosm in the microcosm; Vital centers for concentration; Connection of the Zodiac with vital centers; Crown of concentration; Sequence of numbers; Seven-fold constitution of humanity; Color in the visible & invisible world; Auric envelope; Practical application of these laws.

Ella Adelia Fletcher

ISBN 1-56459-839-X

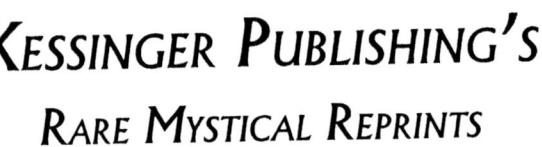

Kessinger Publishing's
Rare Mystical Reprints

THOUSANDS OF SCARCE BOOKS ON THESE AND OTHER SUBJECTS:

Freemasonry * Akashic * Alchemy * Alternative Health * Ancient Civilizations * Anthroposophy * Astrology * Astronomy * Aura * Bible Study * Cabalah * Cartomancy * Chakras * Clairvoyance * Comparative Religions * Divination * Druids * Eastern Thought * Egyptology * Esoterism * Essenes * Etheric * ESP * Gnosticism * Great White Brotherhood * Hermetics * Kabalah * Karma * Knights Templar * Kundalini * Magic * Meditation * Mediumship * Mesmerism * Metaphysics * Mithraism * Mystery Schools * Mysticism * Mythology * Numerology * Occultism * Palmistry * Pantheism * Parapsychology * Philosophy * Prosperity * Psychokinesis * Psychology * Pyramids * Qabalah * Reincarnation * Rosicrucian * Sacred Geometry * Secret Rituals * Secret Societies * Spiritism * Symbolism * Tarot * Telepathy * Theosophy * Transcendentalism * Upanishads * Vedanta * Wisdom * Yoga * *Plus Much More!*

DOWNLOAD A FREE CATALOG AT:
www.kessinger.net

OR EMAIL US AT:
books@kessinger.net

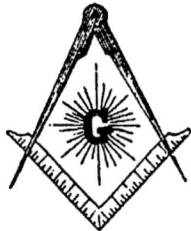

To
RÂMA PRASÂD, M. A., F.T.S.
WHO LIGHTED THE TORCH THAT ILLUMINED MY PATH,
THIS BOOK IS MOST GRATEFULLY
DEDICATED

* * * * * * *

MAY IT IN TURN SHED LIGHT FOR OTHER SEEKERS

"When all the motions of the body have become perfectly rhythmical the body has, as it were, become a gigantic battery of Will."

The body: "A means to an end; an instrument intended for the culture of the Soul."

Rájah Yoga.

TABLE OF CONTENTS

CHAP.		PAGE
I.	"Breath is Life"	9
II.	The Master-Key of Creation	20
III.	How to Gain the Master Key	35
IV.	How to Use the Master-Key	46
V.	The Evolution of the *Tattvas*	57
VI.	The Universality of the *Tattvas*	67
VII.	More About the All-Pervading *Tattva Âkâsha*	75
VIII.	The Specific Influence of the *Tattvas*	83
IX.	*Tattvic* Influences: *Tejas*, the Fire of Life	92
X.	Happiness Vibrations: *Âpas* and *Prithivi*	104
XI.	The Atmospheric Currents of *Prana*	116
XII.	The Circulation of *Prana* in our Bodies	125
XIII.	The Manifestations of *Prana*	137
XIV.	Planetary Influences upon the *Tattvas*	148
XV.	The Activities of the Macrocosm in the Microcosm	161
XVI.	More About Macrocosmic Activities in the Microcosm	173
XVII.	Mercury and the Activities of the *Sushumna*	185
XVIII.	Vital Centers for Concentration	196
XIX.	The Connection of the Zodiac with Vital Centers	208

Table of Contents

CHAPTER.		PAGE.
XX.	The Crown of Concentration	218
XXI.	The Sequence of Numbers	231
XXII.	The Seven-Fold Constitution of Humanity	248
XXIII.	Color in the Visible and Invisible World. Part I.	258
XXIV.	Color in the Visible and Invisible World. Part II.	270
XXV.	Color in the Visible and Invisible World. Conclusion.	278
XXVI.	The Normal Colors of Man's Principles. Part I.	288
XXVII.	The Normal Colors of Man's Principles. Conclusion.	299
XXVIII.	The Auric Envelope: Its Constitution	309
XXIX.	The Auric Envelope: How Affected	318
XXX.	The Auric Envelope: Its Colors	330
XXXI.	How to Acquire Rhythmic Breathing	341
XXXII.	The Practical Application of These Laws	350
	Glossary	363
	Bibliography	370

THE LAW OF THE RHYTHMIC BREATH

CHAPTER I

"BREATH IS LIFE."

IS it wontedness and use, or perhaps, that unspeakably deadening factor thoughtlessness, that has robbed the pregnant aphorism "BREATH IS LIFE" of every atom of its profound significance?

None has ever gainsaid it, yet to the mass of mankind it means no more than if one were to write *omicron mu!* And to that suicidal mania, fear of fresh air and draughts, and its accompanying folly, flagrant neglect of the primal function of breathing, the world pays an annual tribute of at the lowest estimate a quarter million lives; all sacrificed to *preventable* disease! Even without a regret for those sent thus prematurely through the "Gates Ajar," think of the crushing weight of sorrow this entails upon the world! Though not *our loss,* the sorrow affects all within its environment.

But not alone the mass of humanity have been thus apathetic. Until the beneficial cult of deep breathing, a growth in rational doing and thinking of the present generation only, the man of science whose life work is to relieve human suffering equally ignored this flaring torch "BREATH IS LIFE," pointing unerringly to fundamental truths of being, but which throughout the centuries of Western civilization might as well have been a dark lantern. It is my grateful task — nay, happy opportunity — to prove to you that it is a torch of such wonderful illuminating power that man's electric searchlights should pale before it. It was a gain, a stalwart stride in the right direction, to call attention to the error of commonly fixed habits; but all that has yet been accomplished is little more than one drop of purity in a swamp of miasma. Busy people think they have too much to do to give attention to a function they have always supposed automatic, never dreaming of the subtle sources of disorder affecting its normal activity, and as subtly feeding and sowing disease. Also, to make a bad matter worse, in all the so-called "systems" of breathing taught, good, bad, and indifferent, the fundamental principle of rhythmic harmony has attracted little attention, and is rarely understood.

Most persons who are interested in any system

of breathing have become familiar with the term Yoga breathing, yet it is so completely misunderstood that it oftener excites a smile than serious attention; but this is another instance where the precious pearl truth is in sight, and unseeing eyes confound it with a worthless pebble.

All the ridicule, misunderstanding, and depreciation of this cult are in reality due to the fact that few expositors of Yoga breathing have explained either in their writings or verbally to pupils the *rationale* upon which it is based. Reticence on this vital point is due to one of two reasons: either ignorance, or the belief that the age was not yet prepared to be entrusted with a Truth of Life which was till recently guarded in India as a most sacred mystery. But in our day and generation, Occidental peoples accept nothing blindly; all must know the " Why? " and " Wherefore? " We find the answer in the profoundly scientific teachings of Hindu physiology, founded upon the inspirational truths preserved to us in the Tantrik philosophy, and in those sacred Sanskrit writings, the Upanishads.

Only the arrogant egoism of Western civilization has made it possible that enlightened minds could read the Upanishads as they have done for years and overlook the significant facts they contain with reference to the union of breath with life. These facts are the foundation for the deepest, most philosophical, and only scientific cult of physical health and spiritual life; but, clothed in the most poetic imagery, they have been studied, translated, and read for that alone, as curiosities of literature.

It is a deplorable fact that these so-learned minds rejected, without the experiments which they are *assured would verify the statements,* but with cheerful indulgence for the " childish vagaries " and the credulity of those sacred writers who believed them, all these profound truths weighted with the most beneficial results to humankind, and which, in consequence, have remained Occult mysteries closely guarded by the few who understood them.

The forms of Yoga breathing which excite the greatest incredulity, because differing radically from accepted theories of the function, are best described as alternate breathing; that is, through each nostril in turn, the exhalations preceding the inhalations from the same nostril.

This method is profoundly scientific, being based upon a phenomenon of normal breathing almost unknown to Western scientists (eight years ago, I heard of two Buffalo physicians who had discovered it). It is that every human being inhales and exhales for a certain period — nearly an hour — through the right nostril and then all unconsciously changes to the left for a like period.

Hindu physiology begins its surprises by teaching us that with every inhalation through the right nostril a positive electrical current flows down the right side of the spine, and with every inhalation through the left nostril a negative current flows down the left side. The lungs are correspondingly charged with positive, or solar, and negative, or lunar, currents. It is by means of the two currents that all the processes of life are performed, and it is an imperative condition of health that they be equally balanced. Upon their rhythmic and harmonic flow, fed by the breath of life, depends the measure of health and vitality in the human system.

It is of interest here to state that early in 1905, the newspapers chronicled the successful experiments of Dr. Atkins, of the California Medical College, who had discovered, and succeeded in registering by mechanical means, " a positive and a negative electrical current in the air chambers of the lungs of a living person." Thus it will be seen that Western science is painfully discovering the truths which the Orient has had in its keeping since the earliest ages of man.

In two instances I have had substantial proof that something of this knowledge was also in the keeping of our North American Indian " Medicine Man."

But the analysis of breath does not rest here.

Of as vital importance are these facts: The universal current of life, *Prâna,* or vital force, which pervades all space and is commonly recognized in the body as breath (the distinction will be explained later) is compounded of atoms, or electrons, which are differentiated by their characteristic motions into five forms of vibrations. Western science has recognized only two of these subtle ethers, and has not yet discovered their profound influence upon all living things.

We are compelled to use the Sanskrit terms for these etheric forces, which are called generically *Tattvas,* meaning literally a form of motion (Mme. Blavatsky says the *Tattvas* " are both Substance and Force, or Atomic matter and the Spirit that ensouls it "). The *Tattvas* — referred to in the Upanishads as " the five vital airs " — are specifically distinguished as (1) *Âkâsha,* the sound vibration; (2) *Vâyu,* the tangiferous vibration; (3) *Tejas,* the luminiferous ether; (4) *Âpas,* the vibration of taste or gustiferous ether; and (5) *Prithivi,* the odoriferous ether.

These five *Tattvas,* every one of which has its positive and negative phases, mingle in varying proportions in both the solar and lunar currents. In normal health, their flow and proportion varies from time to time with absolute rhythmic precision, every *Tattva* having its period of predominance for a longer or shorter period. If human beings were automatons, the regularity of these vibrations would be as unchanging as the movements of the planets in their orbits. But free will and emotions, every thought and act of man, have their effect for good or ill, and ages ago the Hindus discovered that the inception of every disease is in any influence which disturbs nature's intricate but symmetrical balance of these etheric life-forces; which, corresponding to the elements composing the body, are renewed with every breath and, being elemental subdivisions of *Prâna*, furnish and modify the activities of the whole human entity.

This explains the philosophy of alternate breathing, the many forms of which are devised to restore the balance of the *Tattvas*. It also exposes the error of the statement that, "A strictly well person uses the right nostril by day, the left by night." So far, indeed, from the truth is this, that it would be a dangerous practice, and its exact reverse in a modified form — a shorter period — is the recommendation of adepts in *Tattvic* philosophy. They commend the use of the negative breath — lunar current — at sunrise, and the positive breath — solar current — at sunset; the reason being that the one is cooling, the other heating. They thus impose a certain check upon the prevalent terrestrial influences, while putting us *en rapport* with them, since *two positives* repel each other, as do, of course two negative currents.

In the intense activities of our modern Western life, the positive breath is employed in excess, using up all physical and mental force under the lash of will-power. The resulting exhaustion — sometimes amounting to painful prostration — is because the impact of the positive current has overcharged nerve centers; the human wires over which these currents flow slacken in this condition and refuse to respond to the vibrations playing upon them, so the negative current does not set in. There is discord and struggle in all the atoms to accomplish this, hence suffering. The quickest relief for this condition is to close the right nostril and take a few negative breaths, with deep, full inhalations and slow, restrained exhalations from the same nostril. Only a few moments voluntary attention need be given. Once started the life-current will do its recuperative work.

Beneficial effects are gained by employing the positive breath when going to sleep, which is done by lying on the left side. It counteracts a tendency to an excess of the negative principle in the heart at evening (at which time the negative — or lunar, current is the stronger), and also protects the sleeper from the frivolous and wasting activities caused by the invasion of idle thoughts (called dreams) upon the field of subconsciousness when the guarding mind is off duty. At dawn, it is well to turn upon the right side, but other movements in the night can be made according to comfort and convenience. Nature may be trusted to take care of breathing if we start it rhythmically.

The overwhelming importance of maintaining the equal balance of these two currents will be appreciated when it is known that the excessive preponderance of either causes death; each displaying characteristic symptoms, and causing negative or cardiac death and positive or spinal death. The former is commonly diagnosed as heart failure, and there is little doubt that in many cases the patient could be carried safely through the critical moment if the attendants stopped the left nostril and made the positive current of *Prâna* flow. There are cases where exactly the opposite treatment might be necessary. But if the nurse could not determine which breath was flowing, a few alternate breaths would assist nature to restore the balance.

In cerebro-spinal meningitis, not serum but such care as shall insure the rhythmic flow of the alternating currents down the spine is the treatment the symptoms call for, which agrees with but goes beyond the learned decision that fresh air was the only hope in this disease.

How to direct and control these life currents in manifold ways, promoting health, happiness, and efficiency is the purpose of this book. Those who wish to acquire the power should commit to memory the names of the *Tattvas;* and as a preliminary exercise can practice alternate breathing on a count of four and eight pulse-beats or seconds, for inhalations and exhalations, respectively (that is, four to inhale, eight to exhale), or six and twelve, according to the lung capacity, which should not be *forced,* merely encouraged. Placing the first and second fingers of the left hand so that they can alternately close the left and right nostrils, begin the exercise by a thorough, deep exhalation. Then close the right nostril and inhale through the left; hold the breath for a perceptible moment, then with gentle restraint exhale it through the right nostril; next inhale through the right nostril and exhale through the left. Repeat four times (four negative breaths and four positive ones; eight in all) and practice — it takes but a fraction of time — on rising in the morning, at noon, and in the evening.

The exercises can be taken standing, sitting or lying down. If the former, the spine should be held free and erect; and under no circumstances be twisted or bent from the shoulders; for it is the nervous system which should receive the first and most immediate benefit from the practice. Taken in bed, after retiring, the exercises are very calming and sleep-inducing.

It is by means of these universal vibrations that in actual fact — a literal truth — " The heart throbs of the Eternal Spirit pulsate through " us. It is in this way that we actually live and move and have our being in the God of Gods, the very Light of Light. This *Tattvic* Law of the Universe solves the mysteries of the Omniscience, Omnipresence, and Omnipotence of God, for there is nothing where He is not.

CHAPTER II

THE MASTER-KEY OF CREATION

HARMONY is the least known but the most indispensable factor of health and mental serenity; while discord is the beginning of all *dis*ease, *dis*comfort, and all the family of *dis*organizing elements; the names of which, you may have noticed, all begin with the significant prefix *dis*.

Harmony, therefore, is the law of order,— the normal, natural condition of every atom and its component spirillæ (for which particles science is reviving the name "corpuscles") within the crowning work of creation, the body-beautiful of the human creature, as well as in the visible and invisible world about us; and *dis*cord is the law of *dis*order. To live in tune with the Universe, we must live in harmony with its laws; and "THE LAW OF THE RHYTHMIC BREATH" gives us the master-key to these laws. Studied, understood, and *applied*, no other road leads so swiftly to spiritual consciousness; and at the same time the Law reconciles science and religion as never before. For generations men read Buddha's declaration that ignorance was "the root of the huge poison-tree of mundane existence with its trunk of pain;" but, ignoring his *"Wheel of the Law" in the body*, they have sought for knowledge far-afield, everywhere but within — in self-study and self-examination. And alas! so far have men depreciated the higher self in man which differentiates him from the lower animals, that they have thought to arrive at accurate knowledge of his physical characteristics by submitting helpless brutes to the tortures of vivisection.

When the scientist understands the *Tattvic* Law of the Universe, which opens to him the miracle-world of Nature's forces, he will realize what awful powers of discord he thus sets in motion, powers which, by an immutable law, must return, like a boomerang, upon himself! Then, indeed, will the helpless dumb creatures be freed from man's reign of terrorism.

When we speak of harmony as inseparable from health and all joy in living and doing, we are not dealing with an abstract quality but with a concrete principle of motion underlying the ceaseless activities, visible and invisible, of our Universe — a macrocosm in which there is no "dead matter," but life, life everywhere. To the minutest particle, all is vibrating with ceaseless energy in that mysterious, invisible realm which men are beginning to penetrate by means of cunning instruments devised with infinite patience and skill to supplement the perceptions of the physical senses. Science is creeping close to the long-hidden truths.

One of the recent discoveries is that " This motion is continually changing from one velocity to another." This is the source of that beautiful diversity in unity which keeps us wondering at the infinite variety of Nature's marvelous works, and it is caused by the characteristic vibrations of the *Tattvas*, which are differentiated by form and color, and whose energies can thus be analyzed and recognized on all the planes of their activities throughout the Universe. It is by this means that Hindu physiology has traced their power, office, and effect in the human economy.

We are all familiar with the fact — indeed, every school boy knows it — that our bodies are said to be composed of the four elements: viz., air, fire, water, and earth; yet how many ever think of it as anything but a figurative expression? Now, I am going to show you that it is a statement *de facto;* but how much it shall signify to you, dear reader, depends upon yourself. You must *think*, or it will be barren of results. This caution is based upon experience; for many persons have learned this elemental distinction concerning the nature of the *Tattvas*, and, not applying the knowledge, have gone no further, failing as utterly to grasp its deep significance as in the old familiar statement.

Bearing in mind the previous explanation of the positive and negative breath-currents, flowing in regular alternation through the right and left nostrils respectively, and their differentiation into the *five Tattvas*, we proceed now to an examination of the character and properties of the separate *Tattvas*, and the effect of their action upon the physical, or gross, body.

Âkâsha is the most refined or tenuous of the elements, and on the gross plane of the physical body is correctly classified as ether. Don't let it confuse you when all the *Tattvas* are referred to as ethers, for on their subtle planes of activity they are so tenuous that wanting a strictly scientific nomenclature, we must call the others also ethers. They never, however, lose their distinctive qualities; always, even in the closest union one with another, they retain these characteristics of form, color, and action which betray the presence of the vibration, although every element restricts, and is modified by, the vibrations of the elements with which it is combined. Hence, there are manifold permutations in form and color, producing variety.

Âkâsha is circular or oblong in form, and gives this shape to the orifice of the ear, the organ of hearing, whose perceptions its property of sound stimulates. It is represented as a circle with a single dot in the center and also as a dotted circle; for matter subjected to its influence gyrates with extreme velocity in tiny points that chase one another within the circle. The positive phase of *Âkâsha* is colorless, sometimes described as white, but it is a white pulsating with light; and its negatives phase is indigo, so dark that to some eyes it appears black. In this condition it holds potentially all the other *Tattvas* or elements; and it is the medium — space — in every state of matter which propagates sound.

The study of *Âkâsha* discloses the secret of the mysterious and varied effects of sound upon all living creatures; for every vibration as it passes through the "subtle sound-granules of space" (space and sound being considered interchangeable terms, so closely associated are they) creates its own sound or tone, and registers its effect upon human nerves even when beyond the range of sense-perception.

Thus sound, with its inseparable associate rhythm, is ever building or disintegrating; and is a powerful force that man has urgent need to understand and learn to control, and use with intelligence. Harmonious sounds are upbuilding and life-giving, therefore constructive; while all sounds which we class as noise are disintegrating in proportion to the dissonance and broken rhythm of their crashing and grinding. The suffering such warring turmoil inflicts upon sensitive people is very real; and only more subtle because less perceptible — like the drops of water that wear away a stone — is the effect upon those less conscious of the disturbance.

The vibrations of *Vâyu*, or tangiferous ether — the air — are spherical in form, and its motion is the duplicating of spheres, or groups of spheres. The particular property of *Vâyu* is locomotion, and it stimulates, or gives birth to, the sense of touch; therefore we find its physical influence predominates in the skin which it forms and nourishes. Motion in any part of the body is due to the *Vâyu* centers of that part. It is naturally prevalent in the lungs (or ought to be!) and is regnant in the hands.

The color of *Vâyu* is usually described as blue, but also sometimes as green. I believe the reconciliation of the disagreement to be that blue is the negative phase, and green the positive. In permutation with other *Tattvas* where *Vâyu* predominates we have green-blue, and blue-green, and yellow-blue. When green is reflected upward — that is, the activity is upward instead of downward — it becomes a mirror for the higher force, absorbs the higher vibrations and is then no longer green but its negative blue. All its effects in combination with other *Tattvas* corroborate this conclusion. As we progress to the evolution of the *Tattvas* this will be clearer.

Tejas is the luminiferous ether and the fire element in the physical body, the agent which keeps up internal heat and maintains the body's normal temperature. It stimulates the sense of sight, is therefore regnant in the optic nerves, and must be recognized in the form of light as well as heat. *Tejas* has the property of expansion, and causes the swelling in inflammatory disorders; and, of course, it is prevalent to great excess in fevers. Its form is that of a triangle, its vibrations moving at right angles; hence causing friction which generates heat; and its color is red.

Âpas, the gustiferous ether, is the water element, and in its purest, most subtle state is white or violet in color. It stimulates the sense of taste and possesses the property of contraction. It predominates in the tongue, both in its office as a sensuous and as an active organ, and its semi-lunar (or wave-like) vibrations are the chief motive-power in the production of voice.

The combination of *Âpas* with other *Tattvas* in manifold permutations produces the exquisite variety in vocal tones, gives to them their color, for every tone has a distinctive color, and creates that subtle element which sways the emotions. It is the *color* of the tone, which is a manifestation of its form, that affects the nerves, sympathetically or antagonistically; and a wide field for the scientifically accurate application of the therapeutic value of music is open to the earnest student of the *Tattvas*. The discipline and culture of voice-production in speech itself are thus recognized as of the highest importance.

Wherever water runs over sand, which it throws into waving forms, it furnishes a constant object-lesson on the semi-lunar form of *Âpas* vibrations. The very name wave is a symbol of the curving motion of water.

Last, but not least in this terrestrial life, comes *Prithivi*, or odoriferous ether, the earth. It is the vibration which excites the sense of smell, and its characteristic properties are resistance and cohesion. *Prithivi* is quadrangular in form and, *as do all the Tattvas*, impresses its form upon the nerve ganglia in which it is predominant. Its color is yellow, and it is the disorder of the earth vibration which causes liver troubles, as the yellow tinge of the skin betrays.

For convenience in study and reference this capitulation of the *Tattvas* is given.

	Element.	Color.	Property.	Form.	Sense-perception.
1. Âkâsha.	Ether.	White. Indigo.	Space	Dotted Circle.	Hearing.
2. Vâyu.	Air.	Blue. Green.	Locomotion.	Spherical.	Touch.
3. Tejas.	Fire.	Red.	Expansion.	Triangle.	Sight.
4. Âpas.	Water.	White. Violet.	Contraction.	Semi-lunar.	Taste.
5. Prithivi.	Earth.	Yellow.	Cohesion.	Quadrangular.	Smell.

The *Tattvas* manifest their power in two ways, gross and subtle; our bodies are the gross manifestations of their activity, and through these, animating them and giving them all life, motion, and force, play unceasingly the subtle *Tattvas,* which govern the body physiologically, mentally, psychically, and spiritually, in an ever refining gradation of force, and substance clothing that force. Every nerve center, or plexus, is governed by a particular *Tattva;* that is, is the seat of its special manifestation; thus, though all the *Tattvas* are present, there is a ruling one which is always *in health* predominant.

Now, I neither ask nor wish that anyone should believe any of these statements blindly. Don't accept them because I say they are so. I do ask that all who wish for freedom of mind and body, for health based upon the serenity and confidence that come from knowing the exact nature and action of the agents you are employing to obtain that blessing — I ask you to make the whole subject the matter of serious study and thought.

Reason it out for yourselves. Look first within, in the calm meditation that quiets the troops of idle thoughts which make havoc of our energies and are a never ceasing source of discord; and when you discover that the very name *Tejas* is potent to raise your temperature if you send it with commanding thought to its centers of action (see Chapter IX), you will begin to realize the truth. With the first glimmer of this confidence you will find your attention wonderfully sharpened to the relations of external objects, and no moment of thought on the subject will be fruitless.

In India, nothing is ever told to the student of Occult mysteries which can be learned through study and thought, for speculating upon these hidden relations of the natural forces furnishes the wings upon which intuition takes its flight straight to the cause. In this Western world, however, where the art of thinking is less understood, the student needs some guidance, but the quicker he can stand on his own feet the better. In the physical world about us, you must be prepared to recognize the dominant *Tattva* or the combination of elements in natural objects by the colors. Thus, all the vegetable kingdom germinates in Mother Earth — *Prithivi*, which is *yellow*, and draws nourishment in proportion as it sends its roots deep into her bosom; while it breaks into leaf and blossom and fruit in the ambient, elastic air — *Vâyu, blue;* and from the yellow and blue of its earth and air-progenitors is evolved the grateful, refreshing green.

The *Tattvas* are the artists who grave the wonderful geometrical lines which can be studied in sea-shells. Cross-sections of the shells of nummulites (see Standard Dictionary) show *Prithivi* vibrations. The skin of a rattle-snake is a most interesting study in the proof of the *Tattvic* Law. This creature that hugs the earth and lives in it, is striped down its back with cubes placed point to point, the outer scales of which are *yellow*. *Tejas* is the next most prominent influence, giving sharp points to the scales, and its color is seen in the reddish brown of the darkest scales. Every scale has a mid-rib dividing the positive from the negative. In snow crystals every *Tattvic* vibration can be traced; and, when examined separately, within their dazzling whiteness it is found that all the colors of the spectrum are held latently.

Significant corroboration of Tantrik teaching with regard to the structural effects everywhere in the body of the varied *Tattvic* activities, is found in Bain's description of the nerves. The blue-white matter is in nerve threads composed of bundles of microscopical fibres, of which it is estimated as many as 15,000 to 100,000 are united in a single nerve. The grey-red nerve substance is a mixture of these fibres and *neurons* or cells "*of various shapes,*— round, oval, pear-shaped, tailed, and star-like, or radiated" (*Mind and Body*).

In the *Cosmopolitan* for September, 1905, is an interesting article, "Artificial Creation of Life," by Garrett P. Serviss, the illustrations in which furnish an admirable study of the *Tattvas*. The article explains the experiments of Prof. Jacques Loeb, of the University of California, which have aroused deep interest in the scientific world.

If a copy of the magazine be accessible, notice first the five points of the starfish, which correspond with the five *Tattvas*, as do the fingers and toes of our bodies. Turn next to the large illustration of Eggs of the Sea-urchin; then observe *a*, " Beginning of segmentation," and *b*, " Second step." You will see that the development is by pairs or couples. These are the positive and negative atoms, which acting upon each other evolve every succeeding step.

In *a*, *Âkâsha* prevails; *b*, *Vâyu*; *c*, intermediate, *Âkâsha* predominant, with *Vâyu* and beginning of *Tejas*; *d*, all the preceding with the addition of a strong vibration from *Âpas*, the water element, in crescentlike waves; *e*, *Tejas* is predominant, in which state this artificial creature is said to " starve to death."

Now the reasonable conjecture is that the absence of *Prithivi* vibrations is the cause of the cessation of evolution; and I have had the satisfaction, since making the above notes, of finding the following corroboration of my conjecture: In one of the Upanishads the division of the " fivefold " elements composing the physical body is given according to their use. Water and *earth* are said to be the *food;* fire and air, the feeders, and ether, "the bowl into which all are poured."

It would simplify and facilitate the investigations of modern scientists beyond average comprehension if they would accept as the ground or basis of their researches and experiments the *Tattvic* Law of the Universe. Thus, radium in whatever aspect of its activity is a form of *Tejas*. Every manifestation of heat or light is caused by *Tejas* vibrations. Radium is the highest vibration of the solar current of *Tejas* yet discovered by man; and in February, 1905, Professor Rutherford, of McGill University, announced as a revolutionizing theory the fact that the internal heat of the earth is from radium.

To the "knower" of the *Tattvas* this is the only possible conjecture, for the core of the earth is its solar plexus, and must vibrate with the most subtle form of *Tejas,* sun rays of a power inconceivable before the discovery of radium.

As I weave these notes made seven months ago into this chapter, the morning papers chronicle from faraway Johannesburg, South Africa, Prof. George Howard Darwin's speculations upon "the probability of radio-activity in the sun, which, if proved, will subvert all the scientific theories of its constitution, and of the age of the existing solar system based thereon."

The life-current is more subtle than radio-activity, and it depends upon ourselves to how high power we shall raise it. Never forget that "Breath is the beam on which the whole house of the body rests." If you wish to acquire the ability to apply the Law and use the "master-key," be diligent in the practice of the breathing exercise given in the first chapter. Make the slight change of holding the breath for a longer interval — not to exceed the inhalation — and fix the thought upon following the vital current down the spine; then, while holding the breath, upon the sacral plexus, and follow it upward during exhalation. The length of time must be decided by physical sensations. No slightest discomfort should be felt. Restoration of the balance of the *Tattvas* gives us rose-colored spectacles and all the energy needed to meet life's demands even though they be exacting.

The thought ministrations of Christian Science, Mental Healing, and Faith Cure, which are so "Winged with Power," employ the same force — the only one — and are all manifestations of the *Tattvic* law; for every thought excites a *Tattvic* vibration, just as does the movement of a finger, and the calm fixity and intensity of the thought are the measure of its force.

The throb of the great heart of the universe proceeds from the unknowable primary cause, Divine Spirit, back of all life, and its perpetual source. Its dynamo holds the secret of perpetual motion, fed by the positive and negative currents of Divine Breath, the thought active and thought quiescent or receptive of Him who spake the first Word and declared, "*It was very good.*" And the "Harmony of the Spheres" is no poetic imagery, but describes the rhythmic movements, vibrant with melody, of the Great Breath after the *Tattvas,* by interaction had been evolved, one after another.

CHAPTER III

HOW TO GAIN THE MASTER-KEY

EVERY natural force is ready to work with and for us if we use it intelligently, according to its law. All readers of the previous essays must comprehend now, I think, that the *Tattvic* forces are the active agents of all Kosmic intelligence and energy. Our task now is to learn what is our measure of responsibility for their harmonious movement, and how we can gain the mastery instead of being mastered by them.

In the physical body, the nerves are the lines through which the *Tattvas* speed to their assigned field of influence, and one nerve may carry several vibrations simultaneously just as a single electric wire transmits many messages. The moment they enter the human body, however, the *Tattvic* vibrations encounter the disturbing influences which are ceaselessly arising in the average mind. The reasons for this, though they have so completely baffled the scientist that there are still many who deny that thought can possibly influence matter, are extremely simple, logical, and absolutely scientific. In the *Tattvic* law we find the solution.

It has been demonstrated beyond question that emotions of hate, passion, fear, or a guilty conscience generate poisons in the human system which, when not active enough to kill (the poisoned milk of an angry mother has been known to kill her nursing infant) are the primary cause of many disorders; and they give their distinct colors to the secretions of the perspiratory glands. These effects are caused by the abnormal vibrations into which the *Tattvas* are thrown by the above mental states. Thus with every thought we are moulding these bodies of ours to ease or *dis*-ease.

Every atom, every molecule of your body is as sensitive to the thoughts within (yea, and only less sensitive to those *without!*) as is a feather to a riffle of air. It is only strong, positive personalities who think their own thoughts; more than half of humanity simply reflect the thoughts of other people, for the *Tattvas* carry them to responsive minds. They are the wings of thought.

The usurped over-lordship of the sense-directed mind is the source of most of the ills and sufferings of the body; and its crowning sin and most disastrous menace are that it stifles the soul and prevents its growth through the experiences which should be its daily and hourly portion. The sooner you recognize that you *are* a Soul and have a body (a world-wide difference from the ordinary conception) the sooner you will become conscious of an increased vitality and strength; for the rousing of the soul to conscious activity through this recognition raises the *Tattvic* vibrations to a higher, more subtle plane. The resulting sense of well-being is the proof that you are actually remaking your body of purer materials through the harmonic co-operation of all the elements needed for its up-building.

When once you have experienced the thrill that this consciousness gives you, you will never again deny the dynamic power of thought, nor the deeply significant truth that spirit works through matter.

These physical bodies of ours are always in a state of flux and reflux — like molten metal or plastic gypsum — every component atom taking the form — that is, the vibration, which the thought of the moment gives rise to. Every thought, even the most idle and fleeting which the mind admits to its sanctum, speeds away on one of the wires centering there, to affect for good or ill the molecules influenced by that nerve.

When you banish the army of discordant warring thoughts which sense-perceptions are ever giving rise to, and declare your real self, your soul, the ruler, you are exercising a will-power which connects your soul with the great central Dynamo, the Divine Spirit; and, with channels freed for their flow, streams of vital force will speed over your nerves in full rhythmic currents, which will stimulate all the atoms to harmonious vibration.

Now, the problem before us is, how are we to quiet the frivolous, discord-breeding activities of our minds, so that our souls shall come into recognized rulership of their mundane kingdoms, the physical bodies, and be able to restore the rebellious subjects of these kingdoms to the co-ordinate action which their unity of interests demands? Here is where knowledge of the *Tattvas* is of overwhelming importance to every human being.

We cannot accomplish this by study and reading alone; *knowing* and *doing* are two distinct acts; and it is only by *using* any knowledge that we make it our own. The only road to the conquest and control of these so restless minds is through diligent practice of methods of breathing and concentration; which, beginning by regulating the normal flow of the *Tattvas,* which purifies and strengthens the nerves, then gives us the power to silence the clamor of the senses and, with the soul freed from the shackles of these energy-wasters, to send the vital current wherever we wish.

It is difficult for some to understand how the positive and negative currents of *Prâna* can flow down the right and left sides of the spine and speed over the nerves, since breath, thy say, can enter the lungs only.

The gross bulk of the air, that which inflates the lungs, does not penetrate through muscles, nerves, and bones. But the subtle force within it, that which is life-giving, renewing, and rebuilding speeds everywhere, an electric, vital fluid; and the more rhythmical the breathing the greater the tendency of all the molecules in the body to yield to this current and move in the same direction, which vastly increases the electrical power.

The distinction between breath and *Prâna* is a very subtle one, and most attempts to describe the latter consist of affirmations followed by denials. Even the Swâmi Vivekânanda, who could think so clearly in English that he seemed to have a psychological grasp of Western modes of thought, could not escape the Hindu propensity to strive for the finest conceivable distinction. After saying that the most obvious manifestation of *Prâna* is the breath, and that " This *Prâna* is the vital force in every being, and the finest and highest action of *Prâna* is thought," he concludes by this statement: "*And yet we cannot call it force*, because it is only the manifestation of it.

Other writers are equally baffling, yet this need not give us concern. *Every one who practices will learn to know Prâna for what it is.* To say that breath is " something very different from *Prâna* " is not only misleading but unnecessarily confusing; and in great part the ultimate analyses reached by all these quibblings are distinctions without a difference, a splitting of hairs as it were; for a breath without *Prâna* is unthinkable, since it pervades all space, and has within it the force that moves the Universe and holds the planets in their spheres. Wanting *Prâna* we should not breath at all, and its withdrawal brings physical life to its close.

Prâna is the terrestrial manifestation of solar energy, and its perpetual cycling motion from within outward and back again, supplies the lever that controls the automatic contraction and expansion of the lungs. It is, moreover, the vehicle and stimulator of that thinking principle within us which superintends all the automatic functions of internal organs. The importance of never forgetting the imperative need that the positive and negative currents of *Prâna* be equally balanced should now be clear to all students.

The control of this all-pervading energy, the vital or creative force in every atom is called *Prânâyâma*; and it is in the Held-breath exercise that we generate the will-power to gain this mastery. The philosophy of this is that the force of the vibrations thus concentrated upon given centers, or nerve-plexuses, strikes with such an impact upon the myriad of molecules and atoms as to impart a sympathetic, rhythmical, direction and motion; and, holding steadily to a single focus the customary scattering mental impulses, thus generates higher and more subtle rates of vibration. The higher they are, the purer and finer, and the greater the power of the *Tattvas* which make up the current of *Prâna*.

The next exercise, therefore, for which the preceding ones, besides having their special effect in regulating the vital currents and calming the nerves, have been a preparation, gives precedence to holding the breath, hence its name. The Held-breath is also alternate, and begins like the other exercise with a negative — left — inhalation, closing the right nostril. The usual count for beginners is *four* for inhalation, hold *sixteen*, and exhale, through right nostril, during *eight;* then inhale throught right nostril and continue by same count. A complete exercise is one negative breath followed by a positive, and therefore includes two held-breaths and corresponding exhalations. This is one "round," and four repetitions are sufficient for one practice.

Rid yourself of any impression that you must use force to hold the breath. That will cause constriction and tension somewhere, usually in the throat. You simply arrest the outward motion, and the whole passage over which the vital current flows, from nostril to base of spine is perfectly *free*. If you cannot so realize it, image to yourself an open conduit filled with purest ozone running down through the center of your being. Nothing but vigor can or should radiate from it.

This exercise for *Prânâyâma* should never be taken within two hours after eating, and is best practiced before meals. Four practice-periods daily are sufficient, and the most favorable hours are early in the morning,— the nearer sunrise the better,— at noon, in the gloaming, and just before retiring. It is very important that regularity should be observed in practice. More rapid progress will be made in two regular periods (same time daily) than in many irregular ones. Length of count can be increased from four to six as you gain power; preserving, however, the same ratio, as six, twenty-four, twelve. Upon this point, Hindu teaching lays emphasis.

If you turn the thought inward, following the current down, there will be no sensation of discomfort, oppression, or constriction anywhere during the holding of the breath. Under this mental direction the vital force will surge upon the designated center with stimulating power. The following directions for concentration are to be considered merely as suggestions for practice, and should be varied according to personal needs. During the first round, concentrate the thought upon the sacral plexus; second round, upon the solar plexus; third, between the shoulders, rather low down;

How to gain the Master-Key

and fourth round, at the back of the throat upon the "*nœud vital*" in the great vagus nerve. It is important to concentrate upon the same center or centers in one round.

The solar plexus (back of the stomach and in front of the aorta — the spot often described as "the pit of the stomach") sends out important ganglia through the viscera, and it is to the whole nervous system what the heart is to the circulation of the blood. Concentration in this center not only affects profoundly the whole digestive system — intestinal as well as gastric — stimulating normal functioning of every part, but it reacts beneficially upon even remote centers through the higher power of the electric current thus generated, and strengthens the whole body. Hold the thought while centering it here upon a luminous deep blue disc encircled by rings of yellow, orange, and red. Close your eyes and fix your mental gaze upon the disc. It is a great help to mental control, and you will soon see the glowing colors so plainly that you will not need to imagine them. The whole rainbow of colors can be seen by psychic vision.

Sometimes it is an aid in getting control of the mind to transfer the thought after the first eight of holding to another plexus for the last half of the count. Thus, hold first on sacral plexus, then raise the thought to between the shoulders for the last half of the *sixteen;* and hold on solar plexus during eight, then transfer to the throat for remainder of count.

The downward flowing currents are physical in their influence and the upward flowing are psychical, so it is always best to terminate practice with concentration upon upper centers. Other important centers for concentration are the heart; the tip of the nose; the toes, big and little; soles of the feet when they are cold; between the eyes; the tip and the root of the tongue; the little fingers; and the brain-center, or top of the head. Concentration upon these vital centers is force-creating as faithful, regular practice will soon convince you.

To the invalid who seeks in these exercises restoration of the health and vigor longed for, I give this special message: First image clearly what you wish to attain, and then hold the image steadfastly in mind,— an image, or picture, of health, strength, activity, and helpfulness instead of their enslaving opposites. As far as possible, consciousness of infirmities must be banished. Waste no strength in denial of suffering. It is fearfully real for the time being, but every moment when you can put all the complications in the back-ground, rising to a plane of serenity and harmonious vibrations above them, assists in reflecting better conditions.

This is why we should " become as little children." The child's mind is as free from prejudices and beliefs as a fresh-washed slate from marks. It reflects sympathetically every vibration cast upon its innocent undefiled substance; and it is most helpful when we grown-ups can cultivate a child's power of "make-believe."

We are coming to realize that we choose for ourselves of what stuff these physical bodies shall be moulded, and in the ceaseless activities of our minds determine whether they shall be harmonious or discordant.

CHAPTER IV.

HOW TO USE THE MASTER-KEY

THE secret of all success in every undertaking is concentration of all energy and all endeavor upon that aim. Remittent effort, with many irons in the fire sharing attention and strength, is a wasting drain upon time and human energy; and never, unless under rarely fortuitous circumstances, produces more than mediocre results.

This importance of concentration is well understood in its bearing upon the material interests in life; but its real potentiality is not even dreamed of until, in connection with the rhythmic breath, it is used to bring the mind under control; and, through the mind, the body. This system of teaching the overcoming of the lower self, by no means belittling the body or any form of matter but recognizing the power and influence of every atom, proves to us in clarion tones of conviction the personal responsibility of all who are endowed with intelligence for the perfection of that body through right thinking.

It is by controlling these bodies of ours first, with all their passions and emotions — none of them designed for our undoing but as schools of strength — that we build the ladders which carry us to unknown, almost unbelievable heights of intellectual and spiritual power; heights where we *know* that all lasting, enduring power is indissolubly united with, *because proceeding from*, the spiritual force; and is fed by rhythmic currents of *Tattvic* vibrations of so high and subtle a character that they are unaffected by the disturbances on the grosser planes of being. Only spiritually can we know them; and in rare, exalted moments they give us a perception of the "Harmony of the Spheres." The source of strength thus opened to one is inexhaustible. Practice will give every human being access to it, for the reservoir is within every soul.

The effective use of the master-key is by means of concentration. Only thus can we gain so firm a hold upon the key that we can unlock and open the magic realm of power to which it gives access. The practice of the exercises for *Prânâyâma* purifies the body through the impetus it gives to the expulsion of all wastes, and it greatly increases the flow of the most favorable *Tattvas*, which, speeding rhythmically over the nerves, clear the channels of all jarring and jangling vibrations,— those irregular and abnormal atomic vibrations which cause disease. In brief, this exercise — through bringing the vital force, *Prána*, under control and raising the currents to vastly higher power, more subtle vibrations, prepares the way and the stimulus to gain the power of concentration; for every particle of control over *Prána* is control over the mind as well.

Concentration is the bridge which spans the gulf between the visible, physical world and the wonderful invisible one of Nature's finer forces. It is the first step in consciously exercising the subconscious mind,— the immediate vehicle of the soul's expression. Only by concentration can we quiet the kaleidoscopic flitting of idle thoughts through the conscious mind. Through their train of upheaving emotions, they are constantly beating upon Nature's harmonious vibrations and throwing them into waves of discord. The moment we arrest, through concentration, the energy-wasting activities of the senses, which furnish much of this mental hash, we bring our minds under control of our souls and give our real selves a chance to live and develop the powers which lie latent in every human being, awaiting only recognition and the stimulus of use or exercise to be evolved.

The need for the silent period of concentration is the need for meditation, that men may learn to know their spiritual selves, and gain the peace and strength which can be found in no other way. The man of meditation is the man of poise who meets life's perplexities with the confidence drawn from this unfailing source. In the rush and turmoil of life this noblest part of being lies latent when not denied. The progress of the race during centuries has been vastly retarded by the mistaken attitude towards the soul. It has been treated as a mysterious something, quite apart from practical affairs, which must be "saved" for the future life; forgetful — yea, for the most part ignorant! — that it is ever and always the immanent present which demands the exercise of the soul. By the conquest of self in that exercise — and the first enemy is selfishness — the soul saves itself and grows to immortal stature.

It is the exaltation of the physical body as the mundane manifestation of self whose needs, comfort, and pleasure are of paramount importance that has made possible the development of the modern curse — Sunday saints who are week-day sinners. The man who knows he *is* a soul and that every vibration he sends out will return to him, cannot have one set of morals for the first day in the week, and an antagonistic code governing his business dealings and private life. No one can learn the truths of the *Tattvic* Law without realizing personal responsibility for every thought and act. It is no longer an uncertain belief, or a *creed*. It is absolute self-knowledge, based upon unvarying natural law. And it fulfills the promise that " The Truth shall make him whole."

The cult of the " Power of Silence " arose from the immanent need to save the world from the abyss of materialism into which it has been plunging with its famous seven-leagued-boots of so-called progress. Humanity is just rousing itself to a realization of the depths of degradation to which this mad pursuit of material things as the be-all and end-all of existence is carrying the race. And it is waves of spiritual vibrations, generated by lofty aspirations in the silence, which are thus stirring the public conscience as never before.

From this leaven are rising insistent demands for ethical standards of conduct governing all human relations, and the time has come when these demands can never be silenced till the principle of the universal brotherhood of man passes from theory into vigorous practice, purifying every branch of government — Municipal and National — and elevating all the activities and relations of life.

This is the real Christ spirit which is to rescue humanity from the present intolerable conditions of sordid grind and vicious selfishness; and it is our privilege and responsibility to aid in thought as well as act in this evolution, of which Horatio

Dresser wrote prophetically: "The law of the Christ is the law of organic perfection, the Christ spirit made social is the supreme triumph of all the powers of evolution."

Spiritual thought must descend as a balm to cleanse and to heal the wounds of crime. Not the common vulgar crimes of ignorance or of ungovernable passion which education combats; but the far more dangerous ones — more heinous in the sight of God, more fatal to the soul! — the deliberate, cold-blooded crimes of Satanically immoral intellects which have sacrificed all human welfare and National prosperity to selfish personal greed and ambition. All human moralities melt away before such aims. But they can neither affect nor withstand the force of the stupendous moral wave circling round our sphere.

It is man himself who must ameliorate the present deplorable conditions; he created them — created all wickedness, all crime and misery, through wrong thinking prompting evil doing. There is no wickedness in the lower kingdoms; and through the power of right-thinking man must lift the race from its present state of wretchedness and suffering. He *must* change conditions. Every human being, no matter how isolated the life, can aid the cause by right thinking. It is the quality of our thinking that — *through the Tattvas we draw to us* — makes us what we are, and upon which all our influence depends. Dedicate your daily life to high ideals, and in this training of self-control and self-knowledge your soul will increase in sensitive intuition to all promptings from the creative resources of the Spirit which are infinite.

Horatio Dresser, than whom none has aided more in the cult of spiritual thought, says: " Deep within every human soul there is a dormant intuition which, if it be quickened, will guide us as unerringly as the instinct of the dove, to our home in God" (*Power of Silence*). That "quickening" can be obtained only when we *listen for our soul's commands*. This is difficult in the hurly-burly of life till we have made our minds sensitive to the soul's lightest whisper by wooing it in silent concentration.

Remember that we thus raise the *Tattvas* to a subtle plane, which means increasing activity,— vastly increased velocity. This higher rate of vibrations increases the power of the soul to manifest its control over the mind, in fact, puts the two *en rapport* as nothing else can. The strength which the mind thus gains is shared by every nerve and externalized in the increased vigor and vitality of the body. Existence should be made a joy. Only thus can any soul manifest its highest powers. And to this end the daily life as far as it is under personal control, should be ordered with harmony and restraint. Moderation in eating is important and the purer the foods — the substances furnished for these marvelous *Tattvic* activities — the better the results.

When there is extreme physical disturbance, more especially congestions of any sort, the practice of the exercises for *Pranáyáma* — the Held-breath — would be better omitted. At such times, alternate breathing — on a count of seven for inhalation and nine for exhalation — aids wonderfully in restoring poise, calming the mind, and soothing pain. Hold the breath a few seconds before exhalation, and observe a like interval *before inhaling* the next breath. Repeat six or seven times — that is, from twelve to fourteen breaths. According to need, this exercise can be taken *frequently* — every hour or two — through the day, and is especially helpful at any moment of excessive fatigue and mental or nervous disturbance. It is the sovereign remedy in all crises of heart weakness.

For pains in the back, the Held-breath exercise affords almost immediate relief, and its continued and regular practice strengthens a weak spine more than anything else I know of. It is well to precede this exercise with several rounds of alternate breathing as given above. Do not confound these exercises with rhythmic breathing (fully described in Chapter XXXI). They are remedial and corrective, designed to restore normal conditions. In the well-poised human being, Nature takes care of the regular alternation of the currents.

Instead of counting numbers during these exercises, and especially during the Held-breath, it is best to *think* a rhythmic syllable or phrase, a sacred word or lofty sentiment, the repetition of which holds the attention and promotes harmony. There is a deep significance in this which demands more extended consideration than can be given now. By accenting the first word in each group of three or four (according to count), the mind carries the number without difficulty, rhythm is promoted, and another anchorage is formed for the mind. This affirmation, from Mrs. Besant's *Thought Power,* is an admirable sentiment for the purpose: "The Self is Peace; that Self am I. The Self is Strength, that Self am I." But any thought or word of deep significance to the student will be effective.

In the practice of the exercises for *Prânâyâma* and in the period of concentration following it, the eyes should be closed. This inhibits one disturbing sense-activity, and at the same time discloses to us a marvelous inner vision, whose development, like that of all the senses, depends upon *use*. The first aim of concentration is to withdraw all the senses from every external excitant,

How To Use the Master-Key

for this aids powerfully in quieting the mind. Exactly in the measure that we can hold our attention to a given point, do we increase the rate of the *Tattvic* vibrations, and therefore the force of *Prâna*.

One of the earliest results of regular and effective practice is the discovery that this internal vision looks upon a marvelous realm of color due to the *Tattvas* which we are able to recognize by their characteristic forms and colors. As these vibrations mingle, they vary from their simple forms to those of bewildering complexity, forming every conceivable goemetrical line and figure, and the blended colors producing myriad hues and tints. Many movements whirl around a central dot or vortex, which sometimes gives a sensation of great depth or unfathomable space. This hole, as it were, is *Âkâsha*, the first vibration which was thrown into undifferentiated matter by the great Primary Cause, Divine Spirit — hence, the beginning of the involution of Spirit into matter. Sometimes this *Âkâshic* depth might be described as colorless — a glowing white light — again as black in its intensity, really indigo. These are the positive and negative phases; then, as the *Vâyu* vibrations mingle with the *Âkâsha*, it changes to deepest azure.

Those who have once seen the wonderful play

of light and color within realize for ever and aye that there is a realm where there is no night, and a light that penetrates the densest matter — the light that never was on sea or land.

CHAPTER V

THE EVOLUTION OF THE TATTVAS

IN the evolution of the *Tattvas* we trace the evolution of the Soul to its beginning in the involution of the Spirit. The one is as inseparably connected with the other as are the interacting energies of the positive and negative life-currents; the out-breathing and the in-breathing of the Divine Spirit (or the thought active and the thought quiescent), upon which all life and motion depend.

Thus, spiritual activity is the creator of all things; and the energy behind all motion, without which creation is unthinkable, derives its power from the one source. The first manifestation of that power was positive and negative — the active impressing its thoughts or action upon the receptive passive — and *Âkâsha* was the first *Tattva* evolved by the interaction of these Divine currents of spiritual force. The Kosmic void of undifferentiated matter — the Hindu's *Prakriti* — was formless, and the first need of differentiation was the space in which to create many forms; therefore, the characteristic property of *Âkâshic* vibrations is to make space, and the closer the impact of matter upon the vibrations the louder is the sound of their movement. This is the reason of the phenomenon that Natural Philosophy explains as the denser the medium the better conductor is it of sound.

The homely and familiar comparison (in the *Aitareya-Âranyaka-Upanishad*) by the learned Hindu teacher, of the ether — that is, the *Âkâsha* — to a bowl in which all the other elements were poured, is extremely felicitous and graphic. In very fact all the other *Tattvas*, one after the other in their turn, were evolved and are continually mingled in the spaces of *Âkâsha*.

Âkâshic energy, expressed as sound, has long been recognized as both the builder and disintegrator of form. The wonderfully beautiful geometrical forms into which dry sand, sprinkled upon a drum-head or upon a sonorous plate, will move under the impulse given by musical tones show the ever formative effect of *Âkâshic* vibrations.

It was through an ingenious device of the German philosopher Chladni that sound vibrations were first made visible — *circa* 1785. He observed that plates of metal or glass gave out different sounds according as they were struck at different points; and he conceived the idea of strewing the surface with fine sand, and drawing a violin bow across the edge of the plate, while damping the vibrations at certain points by touching the edge with his finger tips. This established nodal, or rest, lines along which the sand grains shifted, showing the form of the vibrations; and by varying the points of contact, both for drawing the bow and damping the vibrations, a great variety of beautiful figures were produced corresponding with varying tones. It was thus found that a given tone always produced the same figure; so the experiments disclosed an unvarying law of sound vibrations.

Illustrations of these sand forms, called "Chladni's Figures," can be seen in Tyndall's *Sound* and in most text books upon Natural Philosophy. They are of particular interest in our study because they betray the presence of all the *Tattvas* in manifold combinations in the different musical tones, and show how their characteristic vibrations are modified by interaction one with another.

Efforts to establish the laws of tonal color should investigate this field; for color, following form in Kosmic manifestation, is inseparably connected with it, and as invariable as the form. Each may be recognized by the other. Helmholtz discovered that every color has its special vibration (that is, *form*), but he drew the false inference therefrom, that the secondary colors were not formed from the primaries. The *Tattvic* law corroborates the original conception, and by its means the presence of any element can be detected by the known influences, or effects, of the blending of colors.

"In the realm of hidden Forces," every audible sound is a subjective color; and, *vice versa*, every visible color is an inaudible sound. Both proceed from the same potential substance which Physicists used to call ether. Occultists pronounce it, "plastic, though invisible, Space."

The deeper we study the *Tattvic* Law of the Universe the deeper is our conviction that everything in the natural world moves rhythmically. It is only when the human mind steps in with its responsibility of free will to choose the right or the wrong thought and act that life's rhythm is broken and all its vibrations thrown into a discordant jangle.

There is a center of unity in all things,— the ever present *Âkâsha;* and creative power, working in this center, always manifests itself with rhythmic harmony. Holding as it does every form (and therefore, all colors) potentially, *Âkâsha* at all times foreshadows the qualities of all the *Tattvas,* and intervenes between every two. Every progressive step in the evolution of the *Tattvas* is instinct with Divine intelligence, preparing the way for the crowning effort of creation — man with his manifold activities, equipped to conquer and dominate the vast realms of inanimate nature.

Space having resulted from the interaction of the positive and negative currents of *Âkâsha*, there was room for locomotion; and the spheres of *Vâyu* appeared next and began to whirl in the *Âkâshic* vortices, born of the union of the *Âkâshic* currents. Again I must refer to the illustrations of Professor Loeb's biological work in the September, 1905, *Cosmopolitan;* for, as far as that spark of laboratory-created life progressed, it corroborates the Hindu revelation of the evolution of the *Tattvas*, and the law of their several activities and influences.

After *Vâyu*, the next need was heat to expand the air, therefore we find that the mingling of *Vâyu* vibrations with *Âkâsha* produces *Tejas* vibrations of light which generate heat, and which manifest their presence in this dual character. Through the action of heat upon air, water is formed, hence *Âpas* vibrations were the next result of creative energy; and the combined activities of the other *Tattvas* condensed water into *Prithivi* vibrations, completing the primary differentiations of Kosmic matter. Thus, with the fifth *Tattva*, the self-conscious universe, an ocean of subtly fine, psychic matter, came into existence. By successive interaction, following the established law — the *Tattvic* vibrations becoming ever coarser in their descent — the other planes of existence through the mental to the physiological were evolved; till the involution of the Spirit in the terrestrial elements was completed, and the earth with its teeming life whirled in space.

The evolution of the soul thus involved is man's task in his earthly pilgrimage, and it is alone through spiritual thinking and living that he can make that task a daily joy, and feel the exhilaration in facing every duty which more than half accomplishes the work.

A spiritual philosophy of life is the foundation of all *right thinking and living*. In it is found the solution of Ruskin's assertion: "It is only by labor that thought can be made healthy, and only by thought that labor can be made happy." Health is the mainspring of all successful effort, and the spiritually alive soul can command health as the first blessing. It is the natural and inevitable reward of right thinking and spiritual living; that is, living under the direct guidance of the soul.

When we consciously subordinate the physical to the spiritual, all the atoms in our bodies feel an impulse toward order from the rhythmic flow of the *Tattvas;* and even the most rebellious yields to the magnetic attraction and vibrates in harmony with the prevailing rhythm when the currents are fully established and maintained in perfect equilibrium. This is the secret of all the miraculous recoveries of bed-ridden invalids; for in moments of supreme exaltation through faith or enthusiasm, the *Tattvic* currents are raised to so high power as to sweep all obstructions from their path, and to impart synchronous action to the hitherto warring elements, which almost instantly thrills the body with a sensation of strength.

The higher we raise our vibrations through the purifying action of rhythmic breathing and beneficent thinking, the more we shall be in touch and coöperate with the finer forces round about us — their waves even breaking over us — and waiting for our recognition to lift us to higher states of efficiency,— of comprehension, of intuition, of power to think and to do. Spiritual perceptions and spiritual strength make possible a degree of activity — both mental and physical — a power of accomplishment in a given task, utterly beyond the capability of mere physical energy. Work which on the physical plane is effort, becomes a joy and an inspiration when we call to our aid our ever ready, ever waiting, spiritual forces.

It is the attitude of *thought* which makes all the difference, because every atom of energy in the physique has its source in the Spirit. But on the material plane of manifestation, as when we speak of "mere physical strength" or "brute force," the vibrations are grosser in character, unfit material for the Spirit's activity, therefore, lacking entirely the spiritual fire which sustains enthusiasm and gives electrical force to every thought and act thus inspired.

It is this spiritual energy which in rare emergencies and moments of supreme excitement enables people to forget the limits of physical strength and to execute the ordinarily impossible. I knew a very delicate young girl, the accepted estimate of whose strength and endurance exempted her from even the usual exertions of daily life in the home, who, under the excitement caused by a disastrous fire very near, moved several inches out from the wall a bookcase eight feet high which was filled from floor to top with heavy books. It was all that three strong men could do to put the case back in its place the next morning. We can train ourselves to employ this spiritual energy at need, and thus eliminate many of the most trying conditions in life. The wastefulness of common methods of thought is a constant drain of psychic energy which we can better employ.

Every fact that has been stated can be verified by personal experiment, which means persistent practice of the breathing and concentration exercises already given; not intermittent practice when you are reminded of it by bad feelings or when you happen to think of it or have nothing else you would rather do. To derive the benefit, spiritual, mental, and physical which I assume all my readers are seeking, the practice must be regular and at the regular periods — as nearly as possible the same daily. Never let any of the exercises become automatic. Hold the mind to the center.

I have tried to make it very clear that the purpose of the exercises in alternate breathing is to restore the balance of the *Tattvas* and the alternating currents of *Prâna* (positive and negative), the inequality of which is the primary source of all disease. Habitual breathing should be as full, deep, and regular as conscious direction from time to time can make it. Habit is everything in this, and in forming good habits Nature comes to our aid with joyful alacrity. I have failed utterly in my purpose if I have not convinced you that physical, mental, and spiritual harmony are promoted by habits of rhythmic breathing in the purest air obtainable. It need not be cold air to be pure, but it must be fresh, unbreathed air.

Continued practice of the exercises will convince you that you are treading the long hidden, closely guarded path leading to Nature's treasury of secrets. If your interests and pursuits are scientific, before your clearing vision wall after wall, hitherto baffling, will fall, disclosing long vistas cleared and ready for your seeing eyes with assured foundations, basic laws, inviting your fascinating experiments into the myriad permutations of these marvelous forces. Never for an instant are they inactive, but ever building and disintegrating the visible and the invisible universe, involving and evolving through their vibrations every atom therein contained.

CHAPTER VI

THE UNIVERSALITY OF THE TATTVAS

IT should be plain to all my readers now that to neglect proper exercise of the lungs by deep, full inhalations of *pure, unbreathed* air, is a positive self-limitation of vital force which can be justly named "slow suicide." The individual thus living, even under the most fortunate circumstances otherwise, never attains the maximum of his or her efficiency and power, and invites every disease. You thus feed the disintegrating forces with the corruption which increases their activity; and shut out the renewing elements which upbuild, while furnishing the stimulus to cast out the worn out products of physical energy. And this manner of living, which is the confirmed habit of multitudes, is the progenitor of most of the ills from which humanity suffers.

The day is dawning when that infamous old aphorism anent the "ills that human flesh is heir to" will be recognized for what it is, — the hideous subterfuge of ignorance and credulity. It has caused the most flagrant violations of Natural Law, and weighed like an incubus upon the human race, encouraging fear and every other prolific agent of evil and suffering, being a common source of that weakness and inefficiency which produce poverty. Fear breaks down tissue, and disorganizes nerve cells as much as any acknowledged disease. It is only blindness to the latent, the potential, powers within that makes possible the conditions from which a majority of mankind suffer daily. As I shall show you, this is no digression from our subject, the study of the *Tattvas,* but most intimately connected therewith.

When you pray for strength, for health, for relief from pain, do you realize what answer comes back to you from Divine silence? It says to you: "Take them. The avenues are always open to you. Nothing obstructs them but your own will and wrong thoughts."

The moment you think health and strength yourself, that moment you begin to clear from all obstructions the channels of communication with the sources of life-force; for every vibration on the mental plane reacts upon those of the physiological plane. Notice particularly that your very thought is instantly reflected in a fuller inflation of the lungs, which checks the disorder within and improves the vibrations; and throughout the universe like seeks like. Therefore, by a simple change of mental attitude — simple, but oh, so important! — you invite harmony instead of discord, and co-operate with Nature in her ceaseless efforts to restore all the disordered vibrations in your body to their normal conditions of perfect rhythmic balance.

From the ever-blessed moment that you realize your soul to be the rightful ruler of its tenement, the physical body, and bring your will under the soul's control — thereby transmuting it into soul-force — rhythmic vibrations will inaugurate their curative, restorative work. Say in your heart: Peace! Peace! Peace! Ye warring factions! Ye can no longer have dominion over me. I am one with all the power for good in the Universe, and I will admit only good.

The more you know of the *Tattvic* Law of the Universe the deeper will be your conviction of these truths, and of the individual responsibility for health as the first condition for beginning to fulfill God's intentions when he first thought of you. Shakespeare's intuitions grasped a sublime truth. The world *is* a stage; and, like the actors in a play, to each and every one is assigned a given rôle. There is a part adapted to you as to no other; and yours is the task to develop those spiritual and moral qualities that lead to the perfection of your latent abilities, and give you the key, through intuitive comprehension, to the secrets of your strength and your weakness,— both physical and moral. To obey the command,

"Know thyself," is to learn the nature of these hidden forces, the *Tattvas*, whose ceaseless activities, governed or *misgoverned*, make us what we are.

The varying effects of the different *Tattvas* in their activities within the physical body are as dissimilar as their characteristic qualities; and, therefore, the predominance of certain ones, even when that condition is normal, is unfortunate, and their excess is baneful. It is through the freedom of the will that you can control and correct the forces generated in your body, and draw to you the beneficent ones you desire.

The characteristic form, features, and coloring — complexion, hair, and eyes — which distinguish human beings one from the other, are due to the particular permutations of the *Tattvas*, which, on the gross plane of their activities, make up the component elements of different physiques. Their mental influence is, of course, equally important and individual (the physiological being, in fact, its reflection), the opinions formed, the bent of every mind being due to the bias given to it by the prevailing elements, or *Tattvas*.

This individuality, stamped by the *Tattvas*, is determined by the color — that is, the vibration — of the planet under which one is born. This fact gives us the scientific basis for astrology, every planet being the center of a specific *Tattvic* influence just as are the ganglia of the nervous system. This agrees with and explains the puzzling tenet of Hermetic philosophy, "As it is above, so is it below," and shows the close parallelism between the microcosm and the macrocosm. Always an acknowledged truth, modern science has yet to point out the first coincidence. The *Tattvic* vibrations corresponding thus with the planets necessarily vary in force according to their movements; every planet, and therefore the force of vibrations emanating from it, being modified in manifold ways according to its nearness to or remoteness from a sympathetic or a dominating sister orb. Much more concerning these correspondences will be developed in later chapters. It could not be so well understood now. It suffices to state here that every activity in man is a microcosmic reflection of macrocosmic activity.

This *Tattvic* influence is the energy, working by the same law, throughout the kingdoms, mineral, vegetable, and animal of this vast universe. Their myriads of permutations furnish the diversity which charms us, and their invariability that ever-recurring unity of action that baffles the physicist with amazing paradoxes.

In the process of evolution, every *Tattva*, though retaining its essential primary qualities (the properties already described as differentiating one *Tattva* from another — see table of the *Tattvas*, chapter II), combines with the other *Tattvas* in the proportions of 4 to 1, and in the mingling is modified by their qualities. Thus, every molecule of *Vâyu* consists of four parts of *Vâyu* and one each of the four other *Tattvas*, forming a five-fold division; together with two phases, negative and positive, which make up the mystic seven-fold. This number is now recognized in science as establishing the Periodic Law or system, which, grouping elements according to their atomic weight, shows that elements of similar chemical behavior occur once in seven; that is, in octaves as do the tones of the musical scale.

Bearing in mind the process of their evolution one after another from ethereal space to the cohesive resistance of *Prithivi*, the earth vibration, it should be understood that every successive *Tattva*, even in its primary and most subtle form, becomes more complex, for it contains the impress of those preceding it. Thus, *Prithivi* partakes of the qualities of the four preceding *Tattvas*, and adds its own specific property. Two adjacent *Tattvas* mingle more freely with each other than with the more remote ones. For example, *Prithivi* and *Âpas* are more sympathetic and congenial than *Tejas and Prithivi;* and *Âpas* yields to *Tejas* before it does to *Vâyu*. We see this process exactly illustrated in the change of ice (*Prithivic* state of matter) through water to vapor. *Âkâsha* intervenes between every two states, receiving the cancelled vibrations of the element passing into a latent condition and yielding the potentiality of the supervening element; continuing, you see, to serve as the bowl in which Nature does her mixing.

In physics, an important law of motion — known as " Newton's third law "— is this: " For every action there is a reaction, equal in amount and opposite in direction." This principle governs all *Tattvic* vibrations. In the separate *Tattvas*, every atom is reacted upon by an opposite force,— the negative atom by a positive atom,— and when the equal and opposite vibrations of the same *Tattva* meet they cancel each other, and together pass into the *Âkâshic* state. An illustration of this law can be seen when two waves of equal size come together so that the crest of one falls into the trough of the other. Thus meeting, the waves are cancelled and smooth water results. This conjunction, or rest point, is *Âkâshic;* for *Âkâsha* precedes and follows every change on every plane of motion and life.

In the action of light-waves the same phenomenon has been observed whenever a difference of path brings passing waves so that the crest of one set of rays falls over the trough of the other set. The conjunction (Âkâshic) of the two beams of light produces darkness. The interference of sound, as when the condensed part of one sound meets the rarified part of another, and they neutralize each other, producing silence, is yet another illustration of this physical law. It was formerly considered an " acoustic paradox."

These few illustrations show how the *Tattvic* Law explains the most puzzling and contradictory secrets of Nature's workshop. They are given only as index-fingers pointing the way for every interested student to make original discoveries. This, to every real thinker, adds a zest which nothing else can give, and becomes a spur to constant effort and constant progress.

CHAPTER VII

MORE ABOUT THE ALL-PERVADING TATTVA ÂKÂSHA

RECENT scientific discoveries which have tumbled century-honored theories from their pedestals to an abyss where we are hastening to bury them in that oblivion of disuse which the world heaps upon its recognized errors, make it important to the student that a little more space be given to pointing out the interesting corroboration of the *Tattvic* Law which we can find in all of these wonders.

The greatest bar to scientific progress is stated in this trenchant form by Mme. Blavatsky:

"Pure force is *nothing* in the world of physics; it is ALL in the domain of Spirit!" Now, notice this particularly. It is the world of *force* which the modern scientist is beginning to penetrate; a world of such *stupendous* forces as astounds him, and at every step he is coming nearer to the *Tattvic* Law.

The "Forty-nine Fires" of the Vedas are the seven permutations of the *Tattvas* and the two forces, hidden as yet and undefined, behind the positive and negative currents of *Prâna* (7 x 7 = 49). Every one of these has well-determined chemical and physical potencies in contact with terrestrial matter, and a distinct function in the physical and spiritual worlds, with a corresponding relation to a human psychic faculty. To the ancient Hindu adept all these hidden forces were as an open book, and years ago India's *initiates* accurately predicted all the amazing discoveries and inventions of recent years, which have furnished new foundations for science and kept the world marvelling.

Out of the invisible, Sir William Crookes, with his "radiant matter," and Roentgen, with his X-ray, lured two of these "Forty-nine Fires." With the X-ray, the principle of radio-activity which revolutionized science was established; and it paved the way for the discovery of the twentieth-century marvel, radium, which disclosed radio-activity as an actual property of matter. No one conversant with the *Tattvic* Law can doubt that radium and all the radio-active substances can be properly classified among the "Forty-nine Fires" of the Vedas.

In all these progressions and permutations, the higher, more subtle plane, or state, of matter is positive to the next lower, and every lower one is the result of the interaction of the positive and negative phases of the next higher state.

Radium furnishes us with invaluable data corroborating the *Tattvic* Law. But in order to comprehend the velocity of these vibrations (which are ceaselessly bombarding us) and the intricacy of the *Tattvic* permutations, a few words concerning the nature of atoms will be helpful. The word atom is still defined in standard dictionaries, and in text-books upon physics published within the present decade, as that ultimate particle of a molecule which is *indivisible*. In a very slipshod fashion, atom has also been defined as interchangeable with molecule, and, therefore, it has crept into very general usage in the same sense. Although a molecule is described as " The smallest portion of any substance in which its properties reside," it is possible, by means of heat or some other chemical agent, to separate a molecule into two or more particles, called atoms, " and these cannot be further divided " was the ultimatum of Natural Philosophy. Until quite recently, the hydrogen atom was the smallest mass of matter known to science, and, therefore, the accepted unit of atomic weight.

But what says Prof. George Darwin as to this? " It has been proved that the simplest of all atoms — namely, that of hydrogen — consists of eight hundred separate parts, while the number of atoms in the denser metals must be counted by tens of thousands. These separate parts have been called corpuscles, or electrons, and may be described as particles of negative electricity. It is paradoxical, yet true, that the physicist knows more about these ultra-atomic corpuscles and can more easily count them than is the case with the atom of which they form the parts."

Some of these corpuscles move at a speed of 200,000 miles a second, and the unscientific reader will get a clearer idea of their minuteness if told that the molecule, of which they are parts, is so small as to be invisible even under the most powerful microscope. Sir William Thompson made this graphic comparison: " If a drop of water as large as a pea were magnified to the size of the earth, the molecule would appear scarcely larger than the original drop."

Radium gives off three kinds of rays which have been named respectively *alpha, beta,* and *gamma.* The *alpha* rays are compared to the "ions," or tiny particles, which fly from red-hot metals. They are *positively* electrified, and the particles are about twice the mass of the hydrogen atom. These rays have a velocity of 20,000 miles a second, and are constantly emitted from radium in its natural state without perceptible loss to its substance any more than the exhalation of its odor changes a flower. The *beta* rays are *negatively* charged corpuscles, about *one two-thousandth* the size of those making up the *alpha* rays; and, save for their greater velocity — *circa* 100,000 miles a second — are said to exactly resemble the cathode rays produced by an electric discharge inside a Crooke's tube.

The *gamma* rays are not so well understood as the two others, but are believed to be identical with X-rays. Are they not the union of the *alpha* and *beta* rays after passing through the *Âkâshic* state forming a *Tattvic* permutation? A spectrum analysis of the rays should determine this. The spectrum of every substance and element reveals its *Tattvic* nature by means of the prevalent color, or colors; and the greater the heat to which the matter is subjected the nearer it approaches its solar, instead of terrestrial, state.

Âkâsha is well-named the " all-pervading *Tattva.*" In chemical changes of one state of matter into another, you have been shown in these illustrations not only that *Âkâsha* intervenes, but how it acts; that it is the substratum, or base (in all phenomena or paradoxes) which baffles the scientist. As in things external, so it is within; and your observation of natural phenomena will aid vastly in the understanding of your own microcosm, wherein the *Tattvic* Law comes under the influence of your thoughts and will-power, and the currents of *Prâna* may thereby be thrown entirely out of rhythmic balance.

In consequence of its universal prevalence normally, it is not surprising to learn that the excess of *Âkâsha* is disastrous, and according to the phase of its activity causes discomfort or misfortune. Among the traits and emotions which give evidence of this predominance or excess are forgetfulness, covetousness, and obstinacy (headiness), and blindness and unreason in matters concerning the affections. Emotions of repulsion, shame, and fear are due to the same source; and the tremor which shakes fear-stricken people comes from hollows in the veins caused by *Âkâshic* vibrations in excess. To this effect is due the physical and mental tension which so unnerve the victim.

"The remedy," do you ask? What is free will for, if not to give us power to choose our thoughts and the deeds resulting therefrom? The "bliss" of ignorance is that we are not to blame if we do not know the error of certain thoughts and actions. Invariably we must suffer both mentally and physically for such error; but only knowledge, bringing power, brings also responsibility. Never forget that it is the *form* of motion that causes the state, and that form can therefore change it.

A caution is necessary here: It is impossible to energize the nerves when they are strained by constant tension. Paradoxical as it is these two conditions are often confounded, but there is a marked distinction between tensing and energizing the nerves. The accepted theory of tension considered mechanically — as of a wire or rope — is

The All-Pervading Âkâsha

to put all the strain upon it that it will bear. Nerve- and muscle-tension wears people tremendously because it is a stretching, straining, and sundering of atoms one from another which breaks down structure physiologically. In concentration of energy — as in the Held-breath exercise — the reverse is the condition. The atoms are compacted closer and closer together, and thrill with the force of unison and the harmony of synchronous motion. Thus the most delicate and finest nerve is raised to the power of a larger one; and the increase of energy throughout the nervous system corresponds.

Face every mental or physical crisis first, by taking a few deep, full inspirations to change the air — and thus the vibrations, that is, the *form* of action — in the lungs; and follow this with eight or ten repetitions of the nerve-purifying and nerve-strengthening alternate breathing, as directed in Chapter IV. While thus breathing, look within, and seek that heart-silence which carries you to the radiant center of your being, and laps you in poise and confidence.

You will thus raise your vibrations to a higher plane, and in doing this you not only lift yourself into a state in sympathy with higher influences and draw them to you, but above conditions where unwholesome vibrations and thoughts (similar to those you may desire to expel) reach you. You are making for yourself a protecting sheath against demoralizing mundane influences of that earth, earthy character which feeds materialism. Sympathetic vibrations are the wires upon which epidemics spread from victim to victim, and commonly that sympathy is fear. But courage and confidence can be made equally contagious. Happy, courageous thoughts draw the vibrations of happiness and courage; and, steadfastly maintained, will spread a contagion of health and happiness round about you.

CHAPTER VIII

THE SPECIFIC INFLUENCE OF THE TATTVAS

IN the invariability of those characteristics of every *Tattva* which differentiate one from another, we find the reason for the force of habits, and the clue to that inexorable law of like seeking like. This law is set forth in the Bible with stern realism, appearing as so manifest an injustice that to many souls it is a hopeless stumbling block.

What are habits? The established periodicity of a certain vibration, or vibrations; for all forces in nature by an inherent law of their being, come back to their source. This tendency in atom, molecule, and cell to repetition of motion is due to the unvarying law of rhythm. All examinations of molecules prove that their movements are periodical, and when normal rhythmical. All life is a matter of vibration, every act, every thought, is a *Tattvic* vibration,— and once a given vibration has occurred, not only is it apt to recur, *come back to its source,* but every repetition increases that liability and its facility of action, because, it cuts deeper its channel through the directing brain or nerve substance. The great law of rhythm is the director, incentive, or cause of all automatisms. For this reason, also, consonance of action draws similar vibrations together. The way is made and invites that vibration.

Thus, on the mental plane, similar thoughts flash from one receptive mind to another as the needle is drawn to a magnet. On the gross material plane, water mingles with water, oil with oil; and every one knows how all tangible things of like nature are drawn together, and similar events occur in groups whether they be tragedies or festivals. But knowledge of the underlying cause puts in our hands a weapon of defence against the seeming cruelty and hardship of this law. We must ban the thoughts which cut the channels for unfavorable vibrations, and avoid the deeds which deepen and make more permanent their impression.

Ignorance is described in Sanskrit as *darkness* — called *Avidyâ* — and is considered a very dark state of *Âkâsha*. The gross vibrations have become "set," as it were, through the non-reception of other vibrations — meaning fresh ideas; and as the victim of mental inactivity grows older this *Avidyâ* (uh-veed-yah) state renders it ever harder to make an impression upon such a brain. Every new thought makes a new channel in the brain, which explains the high average of conservatism in the human race. People are prone to follow ruts; it is harder to make new roads, which is evidenced in our idiomatic expression, "to break a road." The fewer channels there have been in a brain the less yielding is the substance — "darkness" well describes it — and the more difficult it is to penetrate it with new ideas which must thread their way through. Swâmi Vivekânanda expressed this in a graphic figure of speech:

"The more thoughtful the man the more complicated will be the streets in his brain, and the more easily he will take to new ideas, and understand them." It is not the mere bulk of a brain but the character of its cells, its atomic structure, that makes the intellectual giant.

This follows the law of the whole physical economy, that parts or organs which are kept in a state of activity are more pliable and respond to unusual demands upon their strength or endurance exactly in the measure that they have been exercised. Nothing in the universe is in a state of permanence or stands still as it were. Everything is either improving, building up, or disintegrating; and the atoms in our bodies follow the *Tattvic* laws of universal motion.

But, *never forget*, you are free to choose what the motion shall be; whether harmonious, building up, or discordant, which is disintegrating.

For the physiological plane is a reflection of the mental plane, and your own thoughts can be made paramount in influence, protecting the body from unfavorable vibrations which otherwise would find entrance. So all-pervading, so deep-lying is this law of like seeking like that we gain in health as we promote the health of others; and our happiness is increased in the direct ratio that we make others happy. *That is the line of least resistance;* and the easiest way to win all benefits, guerdons, or material success whatsoever, is to seek those blessings for others.

The mind which is stirred to emotional excitement by the trifling annoyances and perplexities of the average daily life, plunging into wordy conflicts upon the slightest provocation, is wooing every and any physical disorder, makes rhythmic harmony of physical functions impossible, and invites the disturbance of the *Tejas Tattva,*— a most dangerous vibration when thrown out of balance, disturbing its legitimate functions. Every reaction in the form of hatred or evil — even repugnance of the intense sort, the deep revulsions that stir up whirlpools of emotion — disturbs the balance of *Tejas* and weakens the mind, exposing it to be more easily stirred; for every unhappy thought is responded to by an unhappy, disordered vibration. We contribute our mite towards universal harmony by cultivating indifference to evils which we have no power to remedy or alleviate. Every manifestation of control in such cases, by which we *retain our poise* and, therefore, our judgment, also strengthens the mind and increases our power. The energy thus gained and stored is converted to a higher power.

Tantrik philosophy explains minutely the effect of the different *Tattvas* upon human life, health, and happiness, prophesying good or bad fortune for many of the habitual acts of daily life, according as they are performed with one or the other current of *Prâna*, or during the prevalence of certain *Tattvas*. While some of this detail is more curious than practical, and part of it is obsolete, not applying to conventions of modern life, there is much that is fundamental; much which can be proved in many experiences; and is constantly corroborated in every system of mental therapeutics.

The all-pervading *Âkâsha* has centers of dominant influence in the brain and ears; and there are periods when it is prevalent in the throat, spine, heart, and anus. Always active in the exercise of thought, and becoming predominant during intense mental application and in meditation, brooding and melancholy induce its excess, and, in consequence, affect the general health. Knowing this, we must utilize the normal and fortunate powers of *Âkâsha*, and inhibit its malefic influences by changing our vibrations when they manifest their presence.

The natural corrective of happy thoughts is beneficent because they encourage the flow of *Prithivi*,— the extreme of the *Tattvic* scale from *Âkâsha*. Not rose-colored spectacles but yellow ones should be given to people addicted "to the blues," and they should be kept in the sunshine when possible and be surrounded by floods of golden light, living in yellow-hung rooms. Hysteria and lunacy indicate the disastrous preponderance of *Âkâsha* and call for the yellow treatment, and every influence possible that will reduce the *Âkâshic* vibrations to their lowest normal flow. The consideration of *Prithivi*, which must come in its natural sequence will develop more details.

Remember that as the foreshadower of every other *Tattva* all possibilities can be developed from the *Âkâsha*. That is the form of its mental prevalence. It is for us to choose the ingredients and *do the mixing!* It is the stagnation and misuse of *Âkâsha* which are to be shunned. The taste of *Âkâsha* is said to be bitter, but I believe it can also be proved to be salt. It is the lightest of the *Tattvas*. Taking ten as the unit of *Âkâsha*, they increase in weight by ten in natural order from *Vâyu* twenty to *Prithivi* fifty.

Vâyu is only less unfortunate when excessively predominant than *Âkâsha;* and, as their relations are close, the presence of one in excess indicates a preponderance of the other, or is apt to be accompanied by it. In speaking of the manifestations of *Vâyu* or its centers of dominant influence, the reader is cautioned against confounding the *Vâyu Tattva* with another Sanskrit use of the word which has entirely misled some students. The word is derived from the root *va*, to move, and signifies a motive-power. Certain organic functions of the body, which are considered as so many manifestations of *Prâna*, are generically called *Vâyus*, though having specific names. In this sense, *Vâyus* are nothing more than forces of *Prâna;* or it would be clearer to say they are evidences of *Prânic* power. In only one of these so-called "*Vâyus*"—the function of breathing—is the *Vâyu Tattva* prevalent. To avoid confusion, I shall restrict the use of the word to its *Tattvic* sense. It is much clearer to know these manifestations of *Prâna* by their specific names, when we come to them.

You have learned that the sense of touch is stimulated by the *Vâyu Tattva*, and that a specific field of its gross activities is to furnish the thin, elastic sheath-garment that protects the sensitive flesh,— the skin of the body. The two phases, positive and negative, of *Vâyu*, form the positive and the negative skin, each of which has five layers in which the other *Tattvas* mingle, one after the other, with the *Vâyu*, and disclose their influence by the modifications in the forms of the cells. An illustration of a magnified section of skin betrays all these *Tattvic* activities in oblong, squared, and triangulated spheres and dotted circles. In a single layer of the cuticle, it is computed there are a billion scale-like cells to the square inch.

Every movement of the body is a manifestation of *Vâyu*, and acts of levitation are exhibitions of supreme mastery of this *Tattva*. It is more than probable that it is an excess of *Vâyu* which gives people sometimes in dreams the sensation of flying; and deep breathing when walking almost literally gives wings to the feet, so lithe and buoyant does it make the body.

Vâyu has an acid taste, and the acidity of the stomach which accompanies most gastric disturbances is unmistakable proof that this *Tattva* is flowing in excess. All the exercises in alternate breathing, and the Held-breath especially, are of great benefit in all gastric disorders; and I know of nothing else that can give so speedy relief to intense suffering in acute attacks. Four or five repetitions of the Held-breath exercise are sufficient at one practice, but the intervals of practice may be every hour if the need be urgent. Do not confound *Prânâyâma* with the exercise; that is, do not say you take a *Prânâyâma*. You take an

The Influence of the Tattvas

exercise — the Held-breath — to acquire *Prânâyâma* — the control of *Prâna*. Always clear speaking promotes clear thinking and facile doing.

You will understand now that it is the law of periodicity which makes it so important that periods of practice, both for the breathing exercises and for concentration be observed regularly; that is, at as nearly the same hour every day as possible. Regularity in this greatly promotes the harmony and ease of the doing, and increases the benefits proportionally. No ordinary interruptions should be permitted to interfere with this, especially during the first months of practice.

The attitude of mental serenity gained in meditation upon the Higher Self, when we come into a consciousness of inward power from our union with the great Central Dynamo of life itself, gives us a physical poise which is invaluable in meeting the vicissitudes of daily activities and lessens the friction beyond compare. And the benefit is not merely personal. The serenity and physical harmony of one such well-poised person will impart its benison to a whole group.

CHAPTER IX

TATTVIC INFLUENCES: TEJAS, THE FIRE OF LIFE

IT is only natural and in perfect accord with the harmony which we observe throughout nature that the *Tattva* which puts us in happiest relations with the universe while we live on the terrestrial plane is the earth element, or *Prithivi*. Moreover, the fortunate influences of the *Tattvas* upon mundane life, decrease, according to Tantrik philosophy, in exact ratio to their remoteness from the terrestrial element; and the lower triplicity — *Prithivi, Âpas,* and *Tejas* — work together with paramount influence upon human life — for good when harmoniously balanced, and for untold evil when misused. And this influence is not alone upon the gross plane in perfecting the physical body and maintaining the equability and harmonious functioning of all its organs, but also in subtler ways through the great sympathetic nervous system, which is the connecting link with exterior vibrations.

We are constantly lapped in an ocean of life-giving *Prâna* flowing in full currents of rhythmic harmony from its solar center; but in diseased physical conditions, these currents are beaten back, deflected as it were, by the antagonistic repulsion of the discordant vibrations holding sway over the body and surrounding it with their unwholesome atmosphere. Thus, the Universe of matter, to our vision unmanifested, surrounds us. We choose from it what we will!

If we desire harmony and poise, we must *think* of harmony and poise, for such vibrations do not impinge upon either physical or mental states of heat and excitement or depression and worry.

Here is the place to protest emphatically against the false logic which argues that there is no deep feeling, no earnestness, unless it expresses itself with passion and excitement, and defends the strenuous life as the only progressive life of deeds and accomplishment. At this particular epoch of racial evolution, especially as expressed in American life, the influence of this sophistical denunciation of the good, the true, and the beautiful in defence of the bad, the wrong, and the hideous is deplorable. The intemperance of living which it advocates and extols is a national menace, for it affects men and women mentally and morally as well as physically; and characters deteriorate even faster than physiques under the iniquitous strain after success at any cost.

You will learn in this study of self-development — that is, soul growth — through self-control that all great forces, working harmoniously to a given end, come out of the silence; just as Admiral Togo's fleet sailed out of the silent mist on that memorable May morning in the Tsushima Straits, and gave such an exhibition of conserved power as the world never before witnessed. All that this wonderful self-contained nation, Dai Nippon, has accomplished is an object-lesson of superbly controlled force. She is unlikely to fulfill any of the dire Western prophecies of " yellow peril "— fear of which exists only in the strenuous imaginations that picture the possibilities of power *misused* — for Nippon's *samurai* spirit is not predatory.

Those who understand how deeply *bushido* influences the national life realize that Japan has in this word not merely enlarged the universal vocabulary of expressive, high-thought symbols; but that she has given to the world an exalted, ethical standard of character. *Bushido*, " the Soul of Nippon," implies the spirit of discipline and sacrifice, of gentleness and firmness, of honor and integrity, of heroic endurance and chivalry. All that the Western world can teach Japan of material progress is elevated and transmuted through *bushido* into something which the average Western mind — the commercial, How-much-can-you-get-for-it? mind — cannot comprehend; in which, therefore, danger is scented.

But the whole secret is that the Nipponese have never lost touch with Nature. They have kept close to the soul of things, to the heart of the universe, with senses trained to consciousness of the nearness of the spiritual plane, which the Western people have blindly ignored, when not denied, in their head-long pursuit of things material. Japan's own peril is only from those of her people who imitate too closely Western commercial methods, forgetting the traditions of the past, or never themselves trained in them.

We who have worked so hard and made such tremendous sacrifices of the best things, the real prizes in life, pursuing wrong roads leading to precipices or blind alleys and forming wrong habits of thinking and doing, must now go into the silence to find our moral as well as physical equilibrium; to discover the right path leading to rational living and thinking and the forming of normal, harmonious habits.

It is in the stillness that we give the rhythmic breath of life (ever offering its healing restorative power) an opportunity to overcome the antagonistic, disordered vibrations in our bodies, and draw into synchronous movement — that is, vibration — all the rebellious atoms and molecules which have been setting up independent republics, all warring against one another. The state we woo is inward and individual, and not dependent upon exterior silence although aided by it. As the delicious calm of this stillness in which we try to enwrap ourselves makes its presence felt, a poise and serenity flows over and through us, penetrating every fiber of our beings and restoring confidence and power; but few, even when rejoicing in this new-found strength, attempt to analyze its source. It is the magnetism generated by the rhythmic current of *Prâna,* which, sweeping through every channel, imparts corresponding motion to every atom, as a great tidal stream sweeps through its estuaries with irresistible force, carrying all obstructions before it, and compels every molecule of water to flow in the same direction.

The rhythmic current of *Prâna* coming under the control of the soul-centered will thus affects for good the whole being. When practicing the breathing exercises and endeavoring to concentrate the mind upon a given center or subject causes physical disturbance, it is because this control has *not been gained.* The disturbance is open revolt against control and order. Not struggling but letting-go is necessary. Retire to the silence of the soul on the heights of your being, and reflect its calm upon the mind. Downward, to those rebellious physical atoms the reflection must pass on. It is the unchangeable law. The rhythmic word or affirmation is at such times most helpful. There is a monitor within who quickly takes cognizance of the accent and establishes the rhythm, so that you *feel* every group when it is complete. This holds attention and prevents the exercise from becoming mechanical, in which state the benefit is greatly lessened.

The figure of man, standing with outstretched arms, epitomizes from his crown to his toes predominant *Tattvic* influences in the exact order of their evolution. *Âkâsha* is prevalent in the head which is raised heavenward. Out of this *Âkâshic* bowl of mentality comes whatever of good or evil *our consciousness mixes there*, to be reflected upon the physical plane, and affect for weal or woe ourselves and our fellows; for none can live to himself alone. *Vâyu* has its keenest vibrations in those extended fingers; *Tejas is extremely* active throughout the torso, and has more centers of dominant influence there than any other *Tattva; Âpas* is influential in the knees; and *Prithivi*, predominating in the soles of the feet, maintains man's gravity as his feet press Mother Earth and meet her sympathetic vibrations.

A deep significance is here. The living man is the live cross. It should not need historical proof that the cross is the most ancient of symbols — its origin lost in the mists of antiquity — to convince us that like all symbology it originally expressed the recognition of the Truth of Being. That is, the dual Principle — Spirit-matter, positive-negative — and the elemental forces evolved therefrom, which *involved* the submergence of the Spirit, and out of which the Soul must be evolved. And just as the Spirit in order to manifest laid Itself upon the cross (the first sacrifice), the " spark " of spiritual fire radiating from center to circumference, thereby limiting Itself to the sphere, so the soul center of man is at the intersection of the cross just between the shoulders, where Angel's wings are always indicated; and whether there be winged angels in very fact matters not the least. They symbolize the flight of the soul when it recognizes its own power and freedom.

The intimate relations of *Tejas* with the vital organs, so compactly fitting the one to the other in the torso, makes the rhythmic flow of this *Tattva* in its divinely assigned proportions of paramount importance to both health and happiness. Not only does it maintain the normal heat of the body, with centers of great activity in the sacral and solar plexuses and between the shoulders, but it presides over digestion and distributes the renewing nutrient juices throughout the system. In disturbed conditions it destroys its own work. The positive phase of *Tejas* is manifested in the stomach and its negative phase in the duodenum. Its prevalence in digestion explains the close sympathy between the stomach and brain; for as *Tejas* stimulates the optic nerves, it has at all times a strong influence upon thoughts, and correspondingly suffers as strong a re-action from them. Indeed, no other *Tattva* is so quickly affected by every mental disturbance.

The Hindu god of fire — that is, the power or force in this element, the luminiferous ether — is called "*Agni*," and this word is frequently used interchangeably with *Tejas* to signify the same element; though, in some of the Upanishads the distinction is made of naming heat or fire "*Agni*," and light "*Tejas*." The god "*Agni*" is represented with seven tongues, which of course symbolize the seven permutations of the *Tattva*. There are many references in the Upanishads to *Agni* as "the fire within by which the foods are cooked." The student is bade to stop his ears and meditate upon the throbbing he hears within which he should recognize as the noise of *Agni's* activity; and also as tangible proof of the life and light within which are one with the Spirit Divine, in very truth, not figuratively, omnipresent. On the approach of death this inward noise ceases. The forces of life are withdrawing.

Agni is the name of various plants, among them *Citrus acidus* (lemon) and *Plumbago Zeylanica*, a member of the leadwort family. Other plants are called "*Tejas;*" among them several scarlet-flowered ones; and were we to make a careful examination of these plants we should doubtless find they all possess some pungent or heating property.

The fibrous aril of the nutmeg, known to commerce as "mace," betrays in its red color and its fiery pungency its affinity with *Tejas*, the taste of which is pungent. *Tejas* is closely associated with minerals, and during its flow, according to *Tattvic* philosophy, the thought of minerals and quadrupeds rises in the mind. Gastric juices, lymph, bile, and marrow are in Sanskrit called either "*agni*" or "*tejas*." When people are "cold to the marrow of their bones," something is wrong with *Tejas*.

In all hot disputes and excitement *Tejas* vibrations are disordered and increased; and in excess it becomes the instigator of the most diabolic crimes, blindfolding reason and shackling self-control. In Sanskrit, impatience and inability to put up with inconvenience (general cantankerousness as it were) are called "*tejas*." The word identifies the sharp edge of a knife, as also the point of a flame; and all brilliant, dazzling, glowing, flaring things are known as *tejas*.

I believe the *Tejas Tattva* to be the chief force employed in all intense, effective, organizing thought; and also the space-annihilating vibration which is the mysterious agent in thought transference, and which transports us mentally from New York to Tokyo at a speed that leaves Puck a laggard. This conjecture is corroborated by the fact that the Sanskrit name for the brain is *tejas*. The concentration in the brain of this radiant, disintegrating and transforming force in a state of great activity would account for the vast discrepancy between the fatigue effects of mental and physical exertion. It is well known that the breaking down of tissue in the brain during intense application is so rapid that three hours of brainwork is as great a drain upon the physical forces as a whole day of manual labor.

A logical diagnosis of rheumatism by the *Tattvic* law explains its cause as an excess of *Vâyu* and a decrease of *Âpas* vibrations causing extreme acidity of all the secretions and excretions of the body. The intense suffering in the bony structure arises from the pressure upon these vibrations of the cohesive *Prithivi Tattva;* and the relief which hot baths and inunctions of pungent oils afford is due to the expansion of the luminiferous ether, the flow of *Tejas* being thus accelerated and encouraged.

An increased flow of *Âpas* naturally follows, and this water vibration dilutes and washes away the acid impurities whose clogging wastes have choked channels.

For some years before radium was discovered, the miners working in large Montana mines were familiar with a strange mineral which they were positive possessed curative properties. They called it " Medicine ore " and " rheumatism rock; " and they carried bits of it in their pockets believing it a positive cure for kidney and stomach troubles, "miner's consumption," rheumatism, and some nervous disorders. The mineral emits phosphorescent light under slight friction, but there is absolutely no perceptible heat in it, and the radiance is most brilliant under water.

When radium was discovered, it occurred to one of the miners that the "rheumatism rock" might contain the rare new element, and he induced some Butte chemists to examine it. Careful tests and analysis disclosed a trace of radio-activity, and the mineral has been named "radiumite;" but no one can account for its strange medicinal virtues, which have been substantiated by many experiments under close observation of a prominent Butte physician. It is of course an igneous rock aglow with subtle *Tejas* vibrations, which explains clearly and scientifically its magical curative and invigorating properties. To the underground worker especially is it a blessed boon, supplying him with the life element of which his deprivation of sunshine and light robs him.

You see it is of vast importance to human wellbeing that the balance of the *Tattvas* be maintained, and this is the remedial office of alternate breathing.

It is sometimes very helpful in crises of great fatigue and exhaustion following strenuous exertion, to take several full deep negative breaths —

inhalations through *left* nostril — exhaling *all* through *right* nostril. Hold the breath *in* and *out* while you count nine, and increase this count as control is gained; but never do it to the point of least strain or discomfort. Take the exercise lying prone upon the back, perfectly relaxed, or when walking in the open air.

CHAPTER X

HAPPINESS VIBRATIONS: ÂPAS AND PRITHIVI

THE *Tattvic* Law of the Universe, understood and applied in daily life and thought, makes living under the old *régime* of blind submission to unknown forces, generally believed to be malefic and always endangering health, an utter impossibility,— really unthinkable. And the application of the Law leads òne to spiritual living by as direct a course as the flight of a homing pigeon. This radical change of thought is a regeneration, but concerning the transition, there are several things to be considered.

In this pouring of the new wine of Higher Thought, or Spiritual consciousness, which is the only real life, into the old bottles of disordered bodies, the only trouble arises from failure to *cleanse the bottles properly.* Progress will be delayed as long as impurities of any sort are permitted to pollute " The temple of the Living God."

There are many kinds of pollution, and some of the most insidious society smiles upon as pleasures. Gormandizing, dissipation and excesses of any sort which recklessly exhaust nerve strength, and pickling the body with nicotine till the stale, rank odor oozes from its pores, are of these; and habits which thus ignore the body's need of order, cleanliness, and purity within as without must be changed before the " old bottle " is fit for the new wine. It is a fatal mistake to belittle the body, for it is only when we have, through considering its needs rationally, moulded it into a wholesome, perfect body that we can forget it and make of it the perfect instrument for the soul's activities for which it was divinely destined.

When consciousness, in thraldom to the senses, is tossed hither and yon by fear and anxiety concerning the painful phenomena of physical disturbances, the soul is a prisoner in the darkest corner of the basement, and is powerless to exercise control,— it is reduced to the lowest servitude. But with recognition of the real status of the soul the physical conquest is more than half-achieved. There need be no ordeal of purification when the soul rules; no struggle of contending forces in the physiological chemistry; for as darkness is dissipated by light so there can be neither impurities nor discord when the soul turns on the spiritual current. When there is painful physical conflict, it is a reflection of the mental state,— a half-heartedness and wavering of faith and confidence from failure to comprehend the great truths involved, and hence inability to develop the latent soul-force.

The temptation to indulge in those pleasures of the senses which are physically injurious loses its fascination and is seen in its true light when the soul wakes to its real duty and the consciousness of its glorious power. This is the secret of the wonderful hypnotic influence that " cures " the desperately ill, and releases youth from thraldom to petty vices that have enchained the will and threaten to wreck the moral being. By hypnotic suggestion the soul is roused to consciousness of its power and duty, and the soul itself works the miracle.

Moreover, the soul is receptive to suggestion in natural as in hypnotic sleep, for it is then released from the delusions and illusions of the senses, and is itself in touch with higher influences; consciously, when its aspirations lead it thitherward, but under any and all circumstances more accessible to them. It is not, perhaps, generally recognized that " the night time of the body is the day-time of the soul," which was the creed of Iamblichus, leader of the Neoplatonists. This is the divine opportunity for soul growth — the saving provision or means by which God retains at least a faint hold upon even the most wayward of His children. It explains, also, the inestimable value of the quiet period of introspection and uplifting thought which should precede the laying of the head upon the pillow for the night's rest. Incalculable harm is done to little children by sending them weeping and rebellious to bed,— a sure prelude to restless, troubled sleep, with a sense of injury stabbing the heart and rankling in the mind. It is a preparation inviting all evil influences and repelling the good. Life's cares and the world's travail should be dropped with our garments and we should trust ourselves with happy confidence to the blessed ministrations of the divine mystery of sleep, when the soul is offered release from its physical trammels.

The thoughts which occupy the mind at the moment when Sleep gently slips the cap of oblivion over our brains are of paramount influence not merely upon the rest which should ensue but also upon the general health, because they determine in no slight degree the character of the *Tattvic* flow and the equable balance of the two currents of *Prâna*. *Âpas* and *Prithivi*, the water and earth elements, are favorable vibrations whose flow we encourage by cheerfulness, serene poise, pleasure, satisfaction and all pure forms of genuine happiness. We can thus by governing our unruly thoughts correct inherited surplusage of unfavorble vibrations and furnish the conditions that attract to us more fortunate ones.

Remember always that it is the *mind* which dictates every action that disturbs the *Tattvic* balance of the vital current, and that the endowment of free will makes every human being responsible for the thoughts that supply the impulse. The Tantrik philosophers held the firm conviction that if the human mind were *steadfastly fixed* upon any object for a certain time it was absolutely sure by very force of will to attain that object.

Now, tell me, is there anything new under the sun? I must here enter my protest against this age-honored belief in the power of mind being in our day mis-called " New Thought." Its proper name, giving it something of the dignity its due in the revived cult which is mercifully encircling the earth, is " Higher Thought," as distinguished from the stultifying bondage of materialism. It is older far than materialism (only a passing phase of wayward human struggles to know all things marking the close of the Black Age). Why belittle the golden light of the Truth by the term " new," as if it were but half-known and untried?

The therapeutic effect of happiness has been long recognized, and every physician feels that his battle with disease is half-won when he can keep his patient in a happy, cheerful frame of mind. Yet the vital significance of this favorable mental state has probably never been even surmised in Occidental practice. It will advance the science of medicine (purely empiric now) more than any discovery since Harvey's of the circulation of the blood, when it is known that instead of being itself, " a direct product from blood," as noted physiologists have maintained, the nerve-force (called by them " nervous ether") imparts to the blood all the energy and power it possesses. Indeed, Tantrik philosophy pronounces the system of blood vessels only the shadow of the nervous system. *All physiological effects are the products of nerve activity.* Every atom of energy in the human being is transmitted by the nerves, and the form of that energy and the *tempo* of its vibrations, whether in rhythmic harmony or broken and discordant, is determined by the mind.

Happiness is an upbuilding force only equalled by the sun's rays. It is sunshine in the heart! And it moves with a joyous rhythm that sings through all the *Nâdis* (nerves and blood vessels) of the body. Therefore, no medicine in the pharmacopœia possesses the curative virtue of happiness vibrations; while anxiety, worry, depression, and excitement of the heated flurry sort cause varying forms of stagnation and disintegration, which disturb the balance of the *Tattvas,* compel the flow of those which in excess are most inauspicious, and invite the very discord that fear dreads. Wrong thoughts and fear are the busiest builders of disease, suffering, and weakness that I know of, for they are the disrupters of the physiological balance of the *Tattvas;* that is, their manifestation on the gross plane of activity. It is the perfect balance of the positive and negative currents of *Prâna* which maintains life.

In the well-poised, symmetrical, harmonious life, *Prithivi* and *Âpas* are the predominant *Tattvas*. In temperature, *Prithivi* is next to *Tejas*, and *Âpas* is the coolest of the *Tattvas*, exercising a restraint upon the two heating forces, as does *Vâyu* in a lesser degree. The craving for water when overheated is perfectly natural and can be gratified with benefit only, if the water be taken at a rational temperature; that is, cool, but not iced. *Âkâsha*, says Râma Prasâd, " has a state which neither cools nor heats. This state is, therefore, the most dangerous of all; and, if prolonged, causes debility, disease, and death."

The lowering or raising of the body's normal temperature, a condition always watched with keenest anxiety by physician and nurse, is one of the first symptoms of disturbance in the balance of the *Tattvas*. If, for example, *Tejas* flows too long, it is robbing *Prithivi*, which follows it, of part of its assigned period of activity, and the temperature of the body rises above normal heat; and, in like manner, every *Tattva* which exceeds its regular period prevents its successor from setting in when it should; and as every one has its assigned field of activity,— some organ where it is supreme, some elemental need which only that *Tattva can supply*, —*dis*cord, *dis*order, and *dis*ease quickly manifest themselves. This is the real office of pain, not disciplinary but beneficent; to give man immediate warning when he has transgressed the Divine laws which secure his well-being. When the *Tattvas* flow in rhythmic sequence and harmony, the delicate transition of one into another as they change is imperceptible.

All ignoble emotions, as jealousy, envy, malice, carping criticism or fault-finding, and uncharitableness have their physiological effect in disturbances of the *Tattvas* compelling the prolonged flow of those unfavorable in terrestrial activities, and repelling the joy-giving and health-upbuilding vibrations.

Of all the *Tattvas*, *Âpas* carries the breath deepest, and next to it comes *Prithivi*, which discloses one secret of the inestimable benefit, the revivifying effect, derived from deep breathing, without which these beneficent *Tattvas* are denied their fullest activity. The dominance of *Âpas* in this function is confirmed by the great semi-lunar ganglion which supplies the diaphragm with its nerves of involuntary motion. Any injury to these nerves is marked by symptoms of suffocation (as in drowning), from which the patient sometimes dies suddenly. These two *Tattvas* work together in complete harmony, under direct command from the soul, for the release of the body from the dominion of pain and disease. *Âpas*, the universal solvent, slakes thirst, allays fevers, washes away the germs of disease when we will it to perform that office, and imparts endurance under the privation of hunger and thirst.

The exercise of the Held breath encourages in a marked degree the flow of *Prithivi*, and it is brought into great activity during *Prânâyâma*. This *Tattva* gives endurance to acts performed during its flow, increases the power of attention, stimulates memory, and strengthens the will-power. The prevalence of *Prithivi* imparts a golden tinge to the circle of light about our heads and to the brilliant play of light-vibrations seen within. This inner light sometimes glows as brilliantly as the sunshine streaming through the purest atmosphere. It is a startling proof of the reality of this inner world, pulsing with golden glory, which we penetrate in concentration, when, after such experience, one opens the eyes upon a grey and gloomy sky. This has often happened to the writer, whose gaze, from her study windows, sweeps over acres of house-tops to a hill-bound horizon thirty miles distant. At such times, the external gloom seems the unreality!

Prithivi is sweet smelling and sweet to the taste, while *Âpas* is astringent, salty, and is itself the taster; that is, it stimulates the sense of taste. *Âpas* is the predominant Tattva in saliva, which accounts for the extraordinary solvent power of this digestive fluid. It is gross injustice to the whole digestive canal to hastily cram into it a load of half-masticated food, thus depriving *Âpas* of opportunity to perform its assigned work and thrusting upon the other *Tattvas* an office they are unfitted for. Much of our food is put into the mouth in the *Prithivic* — solid — state, and should be reduced to *Âpas* — liquid — before we permit it to pass through the *Âpas* gate of taste by swallowing it. *Tejas* works harmoniously after *Âpas*, but when required to perform not merely double duty but work it is, chemically speaking, unable to do, the effort generates an overplus of *Vâyu* (see Chapter VIII). Gastric disturbances of the most serious character have often no other origin than this. Sudden deaths from nominal heart-failure have been caused in this way, the pressure of the gas — *Âkâsha* and *Vâyu* — upon the heart arresting its action.

The great benefit derived from walking is that through the exercise of the feet and their contact with the ground we are attuned to terrestrial forces. Not only does the *Prithivi Tattva* in the feet increase in strength, but throughout the body it works more actively in all its centers. It shares the influence of *Tejas* in the solar plexus, and stimulates the wholesome normal flow of this *Tattva* in all its centers. As *Prithivi* is active in the liver and in the lower intestine and kidneys, it can be readily understood that the exercise of walking is an unequalled stimulus to healthful digestion, if we eat pure foods adapted to our physical needs and perform the only voluntary process of digestion — mastication — with the care its importance demands.

Âpas being regnant in the mouth and throat is naturally the prevalent *Tattva* in the function of speech and production of voice. As the semi-lunar current of this *Tattva* passes over the muscles of the vocal cords they are drawn up and contracted. The deeper the curves the tenser the cords, and the variations in sound and tone are due to the modifications of this stimulating *Tattva* through its permutations with the others.

The anatomy of the larynx is a beautiful example of the co-operative action of the *Tattvas*. Five cartilages corresponding to the different *Tattvas* enter into the construction of this marvellous vocal instrument, itself of triangular form blended with crescent-like curves. Be not confused by reading in Century Dictionary that there are nine cartilages. All but the ring-like cricoid cartilage, the seat of *Âkâsha,* which connects the larynx with the trachea, are in pairs, and the dictionary counts them separately, though this is not usual in physiologies. The spherical form of *Vâyu* is recognized in the thyroid cartilage (Adam's apple), upon the action of which the intensity of the voice is determined; *Tejas* influence is seen in the triangles of the Arytenoids, and that of *Prithivi* is recognized in the hardest of these cartilaginous bodies, the *cornicula laryngis.* All these forms are rounded and modified by the prevalent *Âpas,* and throughout the whole body its centers of activity can be traced in semi-lunar valves, ganglia, and cartilages.

Concerning the changing tones of the voice in speech and song and their correspondingly changed colors facts of much interest will be developed in a later chapter. The thoughtful student, however, must already realize something of the *Tattvic* value of an agreeable tone in the speaking voice,— of music in speech. Every word we utter has its effect upon the invisible forces around us. It has been said that " to pronounce a word is to evoke a thought and make it present. The magnetic potency of the human speech is the commencement of every manifestation in the Occult World." Remember the formative power of sound, ever building or disintegrating. It is a stupendous force when properly directed, for the subtle sound-space atoms are everywhere; and pleasant speech is every human being's contribution to universal rhythm and harmony, but it affects immediately and most powerfully himself and his associates.

CHAPTER XI

THE ATMOSPHERIC CURRENTS OF PRÂNA

THE Chinese artist Shakaku, living in the fifth century of our era, laid down six canons of art, of which the first and most important principle concerned itself with "The Life-Movement of the Spirit through the Rhythm of Things." It is this "Life-Movement of the Spirit" that I shall now endeavor to make clear to you, disclosing the subtle bonds of rhythmic influence that connect every human being with the vast spaces of the Universe, and open to him its illimitable resources, if he but use them aright.

The broad and general divisions of influence throughout the Kosmos are positive and negative, and all life upon the earth reflects these in all of its component parts, whatsoever their diversity and complexity. Every human being is an electric battery with the regulation of "poles" and development of power under his own control. The physical organism is an exquisitely adjusted system of electrical and magnetic activities, every positive having its receptive negative, and every negative its corresponding positive; and the harmonious inter-

Atmospheric Currents of Prâna

action of these establishes the key-note of the individual rhythm.

But mark this well. The perfect balance of these electrical life-forces can be maintained only through *deep rhythmic breathing of the purest air;* and I shall harp upon this string till no reader can ever forget it for a moment. Be not content with letting some one else breathe fresh air, laboring under the iniquitous delusion that you are too delicate, "too sensitive to cold," to bear it; but insist upon having it yourself by day and *by night*. Not till you do this can you begin to manifest the real power, mental as well as physical, which is your natural inheritance. The want of fresh air is the father of all colds and most lung troubles, and the increased awakening to this truth is a most hopeful sign of the day.

During the winter of 1905-6, one of the largest hospitals in New York adopted the plan of caring for all pneumonia patients on the roof in the open air, canvas awnings to screen from the wind being the only shelter. *Every patient so treated recovered!* During the two succeeding winters, this treatment has been greatly extended, and with unvarying success.

At the risk of tiresome iteration, I must again state that human beings do not normally breathe through both nostrils at the same time; and the breathing exercises already advised are not an arrogant effort to change the natural order of this life-function, but a scientific attempt to restore it. Nor are they new inventions or devices originating in the Occident. The knowledge of correct rhythmic breathing and of the exercises in alternate breathing which purify the nerves, restore the disturbed balance of the life-current, and preserve the harmony necessary for health, is the common heritage of the East Indian people. Down through the ages it has come to them; and the practice of breathing exercises precedes their daily devotions.

The continued flowing of both positive and negative breath-currents simultaneously marks extreme physical disturbance, a nullifying of life-force, and the Tantrists believed it an indication of approaching death, showing the breaking up of the physical entity.

An ocean of solar *Prâna* surrounds the great orb of day, and it is the particular state of its *Tattvic* matter which sustains and keeps in its orderly rhythmic movements the whole solar system. As the vibrations of the solar *Prâna* approach the earth they are arrested by a broad band of *Âkâsha* which gives birth to the terrestrial *Vâyu*. This forms a blue sphere about the earth limiting its movements. No explanation for this is given, but following the *Tattvic* law the natural inference is that the extent of the earth atmosphere is limited by the conjunction of the solar and terrestrial currents, an *Âkâsha*

Atmospheric Currents of Prâna

always emerging from such chemical affinity, as when two *Tattvas* meet and mingle; and from this *Âkâsha* is naturally evolved the *Vâyu* forming our atmosphere, the color of which makes the cloudless sky blue.

This is all the result of *Tattvic* energy; and we must now grasp the sense of that subtle something which binds the *Tattvas* together and directs their activities, ever carrying them onward, and never arrested by them. This is the spiritual essence, sustaining life from moment to moment, always pouring out from the great Central Dynamo under Divine guidance, and borne to us on the solar rays. No *Âkâsha* nor *Vâyu* can arrest it since they are but forms of its ceaseless energy; therefore, these rays, bearing the gift of life to earth organisms, are merely refracted by these media and pass onward to exercise their organizing influence through terrestrial *Prâna*, a modification of the solar state.

The positive and negative streams of the life-current as they flow about our terrestrial sphere receive their direction — that is, are controlled in their course — by the aspects which the sun, the moon, and the earth present to one another. In considering terrestrial life, the first division of these positive and negative influences is that of the seasons, reckoning the six months when the sun is North of the equator as summer, during which the positive solar current flows from the North Pole to the South, and the negative in the opposite direction. When the sun sinks southward below the equator in the early autumn, the negative current sets in from the North Pole, and the positive current flows from the South.

These two great divisions of time, and of influence upon earth life, are called by the Hindus the day and night of the Devas (or " a *Daiva* day and night "). The Tantrists further divide the month into " a *Pitrya* day and night " according to the moon's phases; the light half of the month (moonlight nights) being positive, or day, to the dark half which is its negative or night. Thus, you see, the positive current — upon the physical plane of life, the sun-breath — is always reckoned as the day time of life; and the negative, as the night time. The positive is the period of activity; the negative of the receptive brooding and preparation, *by rest,* for further activity.

Of supreme importance, however, to earth life is this: As the earth turns upon her own axis while moving round the great life-orb, other, more dominant and powerful, and more constantly alternating influences than the North and South currents are developed in terrestrial *Prâna*. These are the day and night currents controlled by the rising and the setting of the sun.

Solar force is centered in the East, and the lunar, or sun-shadow, in the West; and with the rising of the sun every foot of the earth's surface as it comes under the influence of the solar rays receives the positive life-current which streams westward along these rays. At the same time the lunar, or negative, current flows eastward; and with the setting of the sun the daily direction of these currents is exactly reversed. The sweep of this solar current of *Prâna* westward, being much stronger than the Polar currents, deflects the Northern current in the same direction; and the lunar current has a corresponding effect upon the negative current from the South, carrying it eastward.

This is doubtless the reason that the needle of a compass and a magnet never point exactly to the poles, being deflected east of the North Pole and West of the South.

The quiescent moment at dawn and in the twilight marks the *Sushumnâ* (Soo-shum-nah), or conjunction of the two currents, when *Âkâsha* prevails in the *Prâna*. It is for this reason that the Hindu so scrupulously takes his breathing exercises and meditates during these two periods, believing the influences of Nature to be especially favorable.

During the day the earth is negative, having yielded her positive radiations to the lunar current — moon-breath — of the brooding night. Dawn thus finds her in the condition to be receptively grateful for the invigorating rays of the positive or solar vibrations. But there are high-tides and low-tides of this influence according to the direction of the solar rays; and every particle of organic life upon the earth's teeming surface is subjected further to the influence of minor currents from the moon as she passes from one constellation to another in her eccentric orbit.

This varying strength of the solar and lunar currents causes momentary changes in terrestrial *Prâna* which are reflected in our bodies. It is an ebb and flow, as it were; a forward and backward movement; and it is this Great Breath of the Universe that gives the impulse to organic breathing. With its on-rush we inhale, and the current of *Prâna* is sent to the farthest ends of the gross vessels — the nerve and blood channels — of the physique. The succeeding moment imparts the backward impulse and with the receding flow of the vital current, exhalation takes place.

The throbbing of the heart, its expansion — the diastole — and contraction — the systole — correspond with the flow of *Prâna*. But the rapidity of these inward and outward — forward and backward — movements of *Prâna* varies in different organisms. The influences which establish this individuality, inseparably associated with the correspondencies between the macrocosm and the microcosm, are the subject of the next chapter.

The laws governing the flow of solar *Prâna* to the earth and round about it apply equally to all the planets and constellations, but with this difference: the states of *Tattvic* matter in and about every such center are variously modified and every planet has a dominating *Tattva,* just as *Prithivi* is pre-eminent upon Mother Earth. It is this radical difference of *Tattvic* activity which makes all conjectures upon the possibilities of life upon the other planets absolutely futile, till minds can grasp the conception of other planes of life — life maintained by subtler vibrations, or, in terms of modern science, different chemical affinities — with totally changed nervous systems and physical structure.

The need of the hour is to better understand these earth bodies of ours, these vehicles intended to facilitate the soul's activities; to recognize that they are always in the making, and that influences undreamed of by the materialist are ever active in the making. Life is a matter of moment to moment, of unceasing change. Thought is the great dynamic power which determines the nature of the vibrations we draw to us. Directed by a *soul-governed will* we can make them as harmonious and favorable as needs require. And the deeper, fuller, and slower we breathe, the more do we facilitate these natural operations, upon the perfection of which depends the physical well-being.

Spend no breath in denying evil, but steadfastly affirm health!

CHAPTER XII

THE CIRCULATION OF PRÂNA IN OUR BODIES

THE preceding study of our life-forces has taught the reader what that atmosphere of psychic ether is in which, as even modern science has at last recognized, we dwell. We are now to study the circulation of this ether — the terrestrial *Prâna* — as it enters the body and passes from one vital center to another, working with such marvelous intelligence and system that its component corpuscles and "ions" may well be said to be endowed with thought.

The philosophy of the *Tattvic* Law of the Universe is beautiful in its simplicity when fully understood, and the student grasps the subtle relations of cause and effect and holds in his mind's eye a soul-uplifting picture of the whole Kosmos. But this cannot be gained without personal effort, for the law presents at the outset some facts so opposed to the accepted order of things that it seems impossible to explain the theory in words so convincingly simple as to be comprehended by all readers. It is the truth of being which the *Tattvic* Law discloses, but to understand these truths and reap the full benefit of the knowledge, you must weigh them with unprejudiced minds.

Think for a moment how profoundly the authority of the senses must have been shaken when the first microscope revealed to man the heretofore invisible world in touch with him everywhere, teeming with undreamed-of activities, governed by the same laws as the visible realm, and similar but infinitely finer forces than those he already knew and had weighed and classified! When the microscope opened the first gate into the invisible kingdom which surrounds us, it disclosed also the short-comings, or limitations, of the physical senses; and, with many other marvelous instruments since invented which penetrate and weigh and measure the unseen, the experience should warn us never to deny any new thing because our senses have hitherto failed to cognize it.

Then, too, when difficulties present themselves, it is defrauding self to seek outside help before trying to solve them by real thinking — such mental exercise as will make the brain more pliable and receptive. You can draw no knowledge from any printed book, from written word whatsoever, unless with receptive mind you think the matter over and make it your own. Much study and the reading of many books become a delusion and a snare unless time for thought be given and the mind assimilates and digests the facts. Only thus can we invite winged thoughts of inspiration, and encourage the development of the Higher Self.

Moreover, if you would reap full advantage from the study, a state of mind in sympathy with the subject and matter under discussion is absolutely necessary. Antipathy and antagonism, the spirit of denial, close the receptive channels because blinding judgment and obscuring the intellect. An intense desire for knowledge of a particular kind — especially for Light on the Path — opens the way and attracts the vibrations that lead you almost unerringly to your goal.

Unfortunately, most people face a novel proposition with all the antagonism of previously accepted theories arrayed against it. But you must now cast any prejudices you may have behind you and prepare with inquiring mind to understand the only logical and scientific explanation which has ever been conceived of that most wonderful mechanism, the human body. It is a conception which makes natural — brings into the realm of reality — what has heretofore been considered supernatural, when not dismissed contemptuously as " mere superstition," and lifts the veil from the mysterious relations which connect the human being with the whole solar system, and make the physical instrument a sensitive harp played upon by myriads of vibrating waves.

Tantrik philosophy studies and analyzes the circulation of *Prâna* in the human body from the moment that its two currents — positive and negative — establish their northern and southern centers of influence in the embryo; the northern, or positive, focus becoming the brain center; and the southern, or negative, the heart. The interaction of these two currents working from center to center, back and forth in rhythm with the Great Breath of the Universe, guided, directed, and restrained by the *Tattvic* vibrations emanating from every center of force in the starry firmament, gradually builds up the marvelous nervous and vascular systems connecting these two centers of life, and ramifying thence throughout the human entity till the living temple is made ready for the in-dwelling soul!

Thus, as related to each other, the nervous system is positive and the blood system negative; but the diurnal rotation of our earth affects our bodies as it is itself affected, and gives rise to other currents which divide these systems into East and West, or positive and negative halves. The right side of the body corresponds to the East, and is under positive influence; and the left side to the West, and is negatively affected. Then the correlative influence of all these currents develops in each center — the brain and the heart — a further division into lower and upper chambers. In the northern center we know the upper, or positive, division as the cerebrum (always recognized in physiology as the dominant part of the brain), and the lower, or negative, as the cerebellum. In the heart, we can identify the auricles as the negative, and the ventricles as the positive divisions. Notice that in both centers the positive divisions are nearest the poles of these centers; thus, the lower chambers of the southern center are positive, and the upper part of the brain; that is, the hemispheres of the cerebrum. Put yourself in imagination within your egg-shaped aura and this will be clear to you.

The eastern and western currents of *Prâna* make for themselves two main channels called respectively *Pingalâ* (the positive) and *Idâ* (Ee-dah — the negative), which run down the length of the spine forming the trunks of the great sympathetic system. The spinal canal is the *Sushumnâ*, the conjunction of the two currents where the *Prâna* changes from side to side. There is also a cardiac *Sushumnâ* midway between the right and left lobes of the heart. To all these conduits of force — nerves, arteries, and veins — the Tantrists give the name "*Nâdi*," and for the sake of its simplicity we will retain it. The three *Nâdis* above mentioned are the most important in the body being the great reservoirs and conduits of life-force.

Radiating from both the *Idâ* and the *Pingalâ* are fifty principal *Nâdis*, and these branch into hundreds and other hundreds till 10,100 branch-*Nâdis* are reckoned; and through the ramification of these into thousands of "twigs," the *Nâdis* of the third degree become so minute as to be visible only under the microscope; and the total number is reckoned as 727,210,201 *Nâdis*. Wherever this vast net work of nerves spreads throughout the body there are blood vessels running side by side proceeding from the *Nâdis* of the heart.

Thus, you see, the real force of life dwells in the nervous system, which receives the positive solar current of *Prâna;* while the blood vessels receive through the nerves the negative lunar current. The one, therefore, represents the sun, and the other the moon; but these two phases of life-sustaining matter are merely different conditions or states of the same substance,—*Prâna,* the solar matter; and its manifestations in the body are an exact expression of the terrestrial *Prâna* as is that of its solar source.

I shall also use the Tantrik term *Chakra* — signifying a disc or circle — in describing the pairs of sensory and motor nerves branching from the spinal cord. These thirty-one *Chakras* of the spine are brought into existence by the thirty-one sunrises in a zodiacal sign, and the Tantrists recognize a like number of *Chakras* in the heart which correspond with the sunsets. Animating and inspiring the "thousand-petalled lotus" of the brain are twelve pair of nerves which correspond with the signs of the Zodiac in their positive phase; and, likewise, from the "four-petalled lotus" of the heart proceed twelve *Nâdis* — conduits of blood — which reflect the negative aspects of the zodiacal signs (these can be identified in any good illustration of the heart).

Thus the microcosm mirrors in itself the macrocosm, and every *Nâdi* and *Chakra* therein is connected with the greater sphere by invisible lines of a power and influence that human intellect has never yet weighed nor measured. Although there have come down through the ages hints of these mysterious relations which would not be silenced, modern thought has brushed them aside contemptuously as rank superstition. Ere long all the textbooks will have to be re-written.

Mme. Blavatsky says: "The heart is king, the most important organ in the body of man." And she further states that esoterically it is the "seven-leaved lotus . . . the cave of Buddhi, with its seven compartments" and corresponding "brains;" that is, states of spiritual consciousness. The Hindu *Trimûrti* (Trinity) corresponds in the world of matter with Fire (Sun), Water, and Earth; and is symbolized by the Lotus, which, rooted in the earth, grows up through the water to expand in the sun-warmed air into leaf and bud and blossom. A most sacred symbol to the Hindu, this transition from root to sun-kissed lily expressed to him the evolution of the soul through its earthly physical vehicle to spiritual consciousness. Here, again, we have proof of the aptness of the symbology; for these descriptions of both heart and brain are corroborated by clairvoyant sight, which sees, surrounding both these centers, countless radiations of exquisite opalescent prismatic colors. They circle and return, outlining in very fact the many-petalled sacred lily of the Orient (For striking illustration of this see Babbitt's *Principles of Light and Color.* P. 481).

The sympathetic cords — the *Pingalâ* and the *Idâ* — consist of chains of ganglia which are centers of *Tattvic* influence,— the *Padmas* or lotuses of the Tantras. These *Tattvic* centers are of five sorts, taking the form of the prevalent *Tattva.* Thus the *Prithivi* centers are quadrangular; the *Âpas,* semi-lunar; *Tejas,* triangular; *Vâyu,* spherical; and *Âkâsha,* circular; and *Tattvic* permutations form composite ganglia. It is of interest to record here that five distinct types of cells in the spinal ganglia of our friend, the dog, are known to anatomists, every one of which could probably be identified with the *Tattvic* force therein manifested. Although the record of the human neurons is incomplete, it has been noticed that the spherical germinal cells, " partly for reasons at present not clear, later assume, in different regions, *very different shapes.*" The signficance of this change of form, however, seems never to have been surmised by the anatomists.

In Standard dictionary, under the word "Perineurium," an interesting illustration can be seen of a cross-section of a nerve. There are *five* coils of wire-like fibres grouped together in the general sheath. They vary greatly in size, and every coil has its own insulating sheath, preserving to every *Tattva* its inviolate line, though all run over the same wire, or nerve. Presumably, the sizes of the coils vary according to the dominance of the *Tattvas*.

The *Padmas* of the sympathetic cord are closely connected with all the thirty-one *Chakras* of the spine. Those of the *Pingalâ* are, of course, positively electrified, and they owe allegiance to the brain; and those of the *Idâ* are negative and owe allegiance to the heart.

The movement of *Prâna* through the nervous system corresponds with the course of the sun through the signs of the Zodiac and with terrestrial rotation. As the sun passes from one sign to another, the *Prâna* moves to the corresponding *Nâdis* of the brain. At sunrise, the rays of this localized *Prâna* descend every day to the spinal *Chakra* on the *Pingalâ* side corresponding with the position of the sun in the zodiacal sign. Thus, every *Chakra* in turn, day by day, is the microcosmic correspondence with the ecliptical *Prâna* of the macrocosm; and from it the *Prâna* streams along the nerves of the right side, gradually entering the arteries and veins.

Always, under normal conditions, *Prâna* is stronger till noon in the nerve than in the blood *Chakras*. At mid-day these two great life-distributing systems of the body are equally balanced; and this perfect equilibrium fits the individual for the fullest expression of his physical and mental powers. He is in the enjoyment of the noon-day of his strength. It is most unscientific and a brutal imposition upon the stomach to load it up at this time, when the day's labor is but half-done, with a hearty meal of foods difficult to digest. It is a flagrant waste of both strength and food. Only a light luncheon of easily digested foods should be taken. Especially for all sedentary workers this rule should be made a hard and fast one.

From noon on the blood is the great absorber, and at sunset the solar *Prâna* has passed entirely into the *Nâdis* of the blood. The impact of these positive vibrations has beaten upon the *Tattvic* cords of the various sensuous and active organs until they are weary and have lost the power of sympathetic response to external stimuli. Therefore, the fatigue and lassitude commonly felt as night approaches are perfectly normal, and are

Nature's warning signals to halt, the hour for rest has come. When the positive current gains more than ordinary strength, as when will-power flogs an exhausted mind or body to continued effort, the senses are so over-stimulated that they cease to respond to external excitants, and prolonged abuse causes their breakdown. After sundown, the heart — the negative southern center — gathers the *Prâna* to itself, whence it spreads gradually into the left-side *Nâdis* of the blood, and returns from them into the nerves. At midnight the two systems are again equalized in strength; but at sunrise, the *Prâna* has passed into the nerves and is ready for the daily circuit, descending to the spinal *Chakra* succeeding the one through which it streamed the previous day.

The moon, moving twelve times faster than the sun, is the source of minor lunar currents of *Prâna* that move correspondingly faster than the solar current whose diurnal circuit we have just traced. These movements correspond with the movements of the sun and moon through the zodiacal signs; and their interaction is the immediate cause of the periodical changes of breath. Thus while the sun's rays are reflected in one *Chakra*, those of the moon pass through twelve odd *Chakras;* and the lunar current of *Prâna* streams from the spine to the heart in a fraction less than an hour,— 58 m. 4 s.— and returns in the same time. While it is passing from the spine to the right; that is, from the northern center to the East; the breath flows out of the right nostril and, as the *Shivâgama* describes it, the right side of the body is the " full side."

When the *Prâna* enters the cardiac canal, the heart *Sushumnâ*, the breath, for a few seconds, is imperceptible in the nostrils. As it leaves the heart from the left — that is, moving to the West — to return to the brain, the breath flows from the left nostril. And thus, hour by hour, or a duration of two and a half *Gharis* (1 Ghari equals 24 minutes), the solar and lunar currents alternate; and thus they would rotate, " forever and a day," in agreement with the unchanging laws of the universe, but for the disturbing factors of human will and emotions. But the freedom which has wrought so much evil is simply a power misused. It is even more powerful for good.

The periodicity of special wave vibrations which stamps upon every mind its bias, imparting its individuality, is established at the moment of birth by the *Prânic* current prevalent at the time. But never forget that we have the ability to overcome unfavorable vibrations, and the overcoming develops latent power as nothing else can. Self-conquest is the greatest achievement, and the self-conquest won by the light of the *Tattvic* Law is a process of uplifting development, a growth of soul-power, not of humiliating self-abasement.

CHAPTER XIII

THE MANIFESTATIONS OF PRÂNA

WHAT we know as the manifestations of *Prâna* are the periodic changes of its center of activity from one vital function to another in unvarying progression, apparently regulated in the order of manifestation by the changes in the flow of the *Tattvas*.

For these manifestations of *Prâna* are of course manifestations of various *Tattvic* activities. Concerning this the Upanishad explains: "As the paramount power appoints its servants, telling them, 'Rule such and such villages,' so does the *Prâna*. It puts its different manifestations (its elemental servants) in different places," and they follow in the order in which the flow of the *Tattvas* succeed one another; by the "flow" being meant the predominance of one *Tattva* more than the others. It is not to be understood, for example, when *Vâyu* is said to be flowing that *Vâyu* is the only *Tattva* present in the *Prânic* current; but it is in greater proportion — four atoms to one each of the other four — in order that its centers can be renewed. Whether waking or sleeping, while life animates the physical entity, these changes succeed one another ceaselessly and methodically.

According to the *Shivâgama*, the flow of the *Tattvas* is "Ghari by Ghari" (about twenty-four minutes), one after the other; and the current of *Prâna* is active in all the centers of the prevalent *Tattva* at the same time. This, however, does not agree with the teaching of the modern Guras and learned pundits of East India, but I believe I can reconcile the two.

The *Shivâgama* is none too clear in describing these changes, and the Upanishads are entirely indefinite on the subject. Therefore, it is not surprising that some students have confounded the *Tattvic* changes, or the manifestations of *Prâna* in *Tattvic* centers, with the changes of the *Pranic* currents which are much longer, and this has led to some confusion and diversity of opinion as to the changes of breath.

The succession of the *Tattvas* is not in the exact order of their evolution, and it varies also according to the part of the body in which the current of *Prana* is at the time active. Thus, while it is in the back part of the body on the right side, the *Tattvas* change from *Vâyu* to *Tejas, Prithivi,* and *Âpas;* and when the life-current passes into the front part of the right side they change from *Âpas* through *Prithivi* and *Tejas* back to *Vâyu*. The changes on the left side are exactly reversed, for negative action is a reflection of the positive, receiving its impressions as does a mirror that of the object before it. If we could keep this always in mind it would explain many puzzling things. As *Âkâsha* flows between every two *Tattvas* and is active in the *Sushumnâ* which intervenes between the changes of *Prânic* currents, the time of its flow is broken into shorter intervals; and, therefore, the description "*Ghari by Ghari*" could not apply to it.

It is my belief that the meaning of the *Shivâgama* has been misunderstood, and that the description therein of the flow of the *Tattvas* applies to their changes in the solar and terrestrial currents of *Prâna*, and not at all to those in the human physique. Just as the planets are distinguished one from another by the predominance of a ruling *Tattva*, so also is every species of earth life thus differentiated; and the lower the grade of life the simpler the structure and, consequently, the vibration and the color. This is proved in the auras of minerals, which show only one color, and of the flora and fauna which display more and more complex colors as they ascend in the scale of life.

As you might conjecture from its life under the ground, in the busy ant *Privithi* is the dominant *Tattva;* and the reason the fly goes into hiding or persistently attacks the human being and all warm-blooded creatures when cold winds blow and on raw, damp days, is that *Tejas* is its life element. I have found that the most obstinate nuisance will cease his persecutions on such days if a pitcher of hot water be placed nearby. He will hug it as long as warmth lingers. In the birds of the air *Vâyu* predominates over *Prithivi*, while in the quadruped who clings to the earth with four feet this is exactly reversed.

I have frequently given emphasis to the fact that upon man is placed the responsibility of choosing for himself what shall be the dominant *Tattvic* activities of his being, and that upon his choice depends not alone his own weal and woe but the comfort, happiness, and well-being of all whose lives are connected with him. Therefore, knowing as you do now the terrestrial influences of the various *Tattvas*, it must certainly appeal to you as more logical that some of them should have a greater normal flow than others; and this is exactly the teaching at the present time of the East Indian Guras. By this method, their order is as given above, but *Vâyu* is said to flow eight minutes; *Tejas*, twelve minutes; *Prithivi*, twenty minutes; *Âpas*, sixteen minutes; and *Âkâsha*, only four. As this totals sixty minutes, the rational conclusion is that the exact period is a fraction less and that there is one complete change of the

Manifestations of Prâna

Tattvas during the flow of each current of *Prâna*.

Now, if you remember that five *Gharis* are about equal to two hours you will understand that by the *Shivâgama* reckoning we are confronted with the puzzling statement that there is only one complete change of the *Tattvas* during the flow of the two currents, that is during a positive period when the breath is in the right lung and the currents are flowing from the northern to the southern center; and a negative one when the breath is in the left lung and the direction is reversed, the *Prâna* flowing from the heart, or southern center, northward on the left side. Yet the statement is also made in the *Shivâgama* that "In the left as well as in the right there is the five-fold rise" [of the *Tattvas*]. That the *Tattvic* changes in the world current are "Ghari by Ghari" is my conviction.

With regard to the two currents of *Prâna*, it is significant that the period of their flow exactly corresponds with a twelfth of the moon's eccentric diurnal orbit, during which period there is a marked change in her elongation, or angular distance from the sun, and this change in the wave vibrations is reflected in the breath. The Tantrists believed the lunar current to be most powerful during the rise of Taurus, Cancer, Virgo, Scorpio, Capricornus, and Pisces; and the solar current to be dominant when Aries, Gemini, Leo, Libra, Sagittarius, and Aquarius are in the ascendant.

To understand this clearly we must grasp the conception of the wheel within wheels,— the ever-present positive and negative forces in every division of every activity down to the infinitesimal molecule. Thus, though the lunar current is negative to the solar, it is itself compounded of positive and negative atoms and has its positive aspect. In no other way can we reconcile the flow of the lunar current southward on the right (the positive) side to the heart, during which time the breath flows from the positive nostril. Therefore, in its effects and action, or movement, it is like the solar current, for it is positively electrified. We are simply to understand that the course of the current through the body is influenced by the direction given to the moon's rays from its position in the heavens.

But always the *Rayi*—lunar current, or negative phase of *Prâna*—is the "cooler state of life-matter which is only the shade of *Prâna*, the original state." It "has the qualities of Amrita, the giver of eternal life;" and also, "In the left *Nâdi*, the appearance of the breath is that of the Amrita (nectar); it is the great nourisher of the world."

On the first lunar day — that is, the first day of the "bright fortnight," or moonlight nights — the lunar current, which is then the stronger, is said to flow at the rising of the sun, and during the dark fortnight the solar current comes in first, the currents alternating one after the other as previously described. In spite of this normal order, however, Tantrik philosophy teaches that "It confers groups of good qualities" to cause the negative breath to flow at sunrise and the positive breath at sundown. Any electrician should understand the *rationale* of this, for it puts the body in a receptive condition towards the terrestrial *Prâna*, which is at the maximum of its positive phase at sunrise. If it is the normal condition for the lunar current to come in first during the bright fortnight, we need seek no further reason for its being considered the most fortunate half of the month, especially for women, who are the negative half of humanity.

The most important of the manifestations of *Prâna* are five in number, though the Hindu proness to the ultimate analysis rests not till it enumerates ten of these forces, or so-called *Vâyus*. But as the five minor ones are but modifications of the others, signs as it were of their activities, we will confine our examination to those governing organic functions.

The first is the act of breathing, and as this function is the key to the changes of the life-current, it bears the same name and is identified as *Prâna*, being, says Râma Prasâd, "that manifestation of the life-coil which draws atmospheric air from without into the system." *Vâyu* is the prevalent *Tattva*, and the right lung is the seat of its positive phase, and the left, of the negative. The pulmonary circulation of blood in the upper *Chakra* (the cavity of the chest) is positive to that in the lower *Chakra* (below the diaphragm), but also arterial blood in both *Chakras*, or systems of circulation, is positive to the negative veins. The capillaries are the *Sushumnâ* of the vascular system. Thus, again, you find the wheel within wheel.

The second manifestation of *Prâna* is *Samâna* which governs the processes of digestion and assimilation, carrying the nutrient juices where needed. *Tejas* is the ruling *Tattva*, and the stomach and navel the seats of its positive phase, while the negative phase is active in the duodenum. *Apâna*, the third manifestation, governs the excretory functions, in which *Prithivi* predominates; the positive phase working in the long intestine, and the negative, in the kidneys. As *Apâna* is said to throw "from inside, out of the system, things which are not needed there," it is reasonable to conclude that the function of *Prithivi* in both skin and lungs is excretory, and that perspiration is also a manifestation of *Apâna*.

Vyâna, the fourth manifestation, is the seat of *Âpas*, and is present all over the body, being that force, which, during life keeps all parts in perfect shape and resists breaking down and disintegration. This preponderance of *Âpas* — five-sixths of the human body is water — can be traced throughout the physical structure, its seats of influence being more clearly defined anatomically than those of any other *Tattva*. The semi-lunar valves in arteries and veins are among these.

The fifth manifestation is *Udâna*, the seat of *Âkâsha*. It is the power which inclines the life-forces back to the centers — northern or southern — and is regnant therefore in the spine and heart, and also in the throat. A lump in the throat, when the breath catches and almost goes, after a quick run, proclaims the presence of *Udâna*, and this manifestation is dangerous. It is evidence of the excess of one current, and if it passes to a certain delicate line beyond the ordinary limit, the opposite current fails to react, *Prâna* remains in the *Sushumnâ*, and death results. These are the moments when life hangs by a thread, so delicate is the balance. To stimulate the opposite current to flow is the need at this critical moment, and probably in most cases it is the positive current which has done the mischief.

Whole books of the Upanishads are devoted to poetical descriptions of these manifestations of *Prâna*, imagination revelling in depicting their power. *Prâna* is usually described as declaring "itself five-fold" through "unfolding" the various elements, or *Tattvas*, in these several manifestations. There are said to be "five gates to the heart," for the Devas, or senses (remember that every sense corresponds to a special *Tattva* which stimulates its activity), and the heart is the ruler of the sensuous and active organs. The heart receives impressions from the positive *Prâna*, and it is the nature of the heart's reflection of these upon which human actions and the work of the world depend. The eastern gate is *Prâna*, manifested in "up-breathing." *Apâna*, the western gate, is described as down-breathing, and the deity that exists in the earth (in modern phraseology, gravity) is there to support man's *Apâna*, ever attracting its activities downwards.

Samâna, the northern gate, is described as on-breathing, because it impels the grosser materials of food to the *Apâna*, and conveys the finer and more subtle nutriment to the limbs. *Vyâna* is the southern gate, and, pervading the blood-*Nâdis*, is recognized as back-breathing. *Udâna* is called the upper gate, and distinguished as out-breathing, being most perceptible in the throat. Now, this upward impulse has its normal beneficent phase, encouraging "growth, lightness and agility," and it is evil only when the currents are unbalanced; for the *Tattvic* Law of Harmony requires that these two vital creative forces be equally active, but alternately dominate one another.

As these manifestations change from one to another the state of *Sushumnâ* intervenes; therefore, the rays of *Sushumnâ* extend all over the body midway between the positive and negative *Nâdis*, and are the medium by which the *Prâna* passes back and forth from the positive to the negative parts of the body and *vice versa*.

The rule holds good to all eternity that like seeks like. You must think in harmony with the purest vibrations of the external world, if you would reap the benefit of your kinship with all good and all power in the Universe. Understand well and clearly this fact: The very ability to think at all implies the freedom to use the power beneficently instead of harmfully,— to change your thoughts from one thing to another as easily as you do your garments. Nothing is impossible to the soul-directed thought; failure is through want of faith, of fixedness of purpose and aim; success is in direct proportion to the unswerving trust of our belief. It is we who fail; never the law! Our very failures testify to that.

CHAPTER XIV

PLANETARY INFLUENCES UPON THE TATTVAS

WE have heretofore considered the regular, normal order of the solar and lunar currents of *Prâna*, and it should be clearly understood by this time that the *Tattvic* state of these currents is a most important factor in determining the beneficial effects upon the whole physical being of their even, balanced flow in deep, full rhythmical breathing.

The paramount influence affecting this comes from the planets, every one of which establishes its own currents in the organism, determined in degree and kind by the planets' position in the firmament and consequent relation with all other planets. It is the strength of these currents, varying in different people, which distinguishes the individualized, local *Prâna* from the universal terrestrial *Prâna*. In this fact we find corroboration of all that astrology claims concerning the planetary influences at the moment of birth upon human life and character.

There are seven descriptions of life-currents,

corresponding exactly with the planets of the solar system and influenced by them, which flow around the spinal *Chakras*, every *Chakra* being itself, *in the activities therein centered*, a minature copy of the Zodiac with divisions of influence corresponding to its heavenly signs. Several of these currents, or even all, may be passing along at the same time over the same nerve and around the same *Chakra*, just as varying electric currents pass simultaneously over the same wire. The multitudinous fibers in a single nerve prevent any " interference." But every *Tattva* will be more active in certain divisions of the *Chakra* according to the position in the Zodiac of the planetary influence; for the vibrations of the microcosm correspond with those of the macrocosm.

These seven variations are all to be understood as *Tattvic* modifications of *Prâna*, and they would flow on forever and aye within the body as without in undisturbed harmony when Nature is serene, and affected by her storms only when in planetary, or *Tattvic* sympathy with them, but for the erratic working of human free will. As already stated many times, all disease is the result of disturbances in the regular balance of the positive and negative, or solar and lunar, currents of *Prâna*, and of the normal flow of the *Tattvas;* and human errors, emotions, and deeds are the most common disturbing factors. But the changes thus injected into the localized, or individualized, *Prâna* prove to us as nothing else can the dynamic power of thought, *itself manipulating and disturbing these forces and therefore superior to them;* and disclose to the spiritually alive soul glimpses of limitless realms for conquest.

To the materialist these realms of power are a sealed book, and will forever remain beyond his vision. He is the victim of self-limitation! They are accessible only to the soul-directed will, which, governing thought, chooses the right path and carries consciousness to higher planes of harmonic vibrations. The human instrument is thus tuned to purer and higher influences.

An ocean of thought-vibrations is beating upon our brains every instant, seeking sympathetic vibrations upon which to impinge. This is the secret of the same thought flashing through many brains *under the same Tattvic influence* at the same time. While this *Tattvic* (or planetary) influence determines the thoughts and the deeds of the drifters and all in negative — that is, receptive — conditions, OURS IS THE POWER TO CHOOSE THE THOUGHT. The free will that is a peril is also the greatest blessing, putting in our grasp the ever-ready means to overcome physical evils; and the needs of the hour are ethical training in choice, and the *education of the will*. Evil seeks evil with a marvellous power of accretion and disturbance, but think not for a moment that all good is not even more powerful. The one corresponds to darkness, the other to light; the one is disintegrating, the other upbuilding and renewing. "There is in things evil an element of self-destruction, in the operation of which lies the safety of the Universe" (*The Perfect Way*, p. 189).

Thus the *Tattvic* state of *Prâna* in every human being is determined by the position and strength of the various local currents. Color in different plexuses varies from moment to moment as the *Tattvic* currents change and according to the flow of the *Prânic* current, the state of which — positive or negative — modifies the prevalent color. The negative current of *Prâna* is said to be pure white, and the positive is tinged with red,— sometimes described as rose-color. This agrees perfectly with the color of the nerves, the sensory (afferent and posterior), which are the negative ones, being bluish-white; and the motor (efferent and anterior), are reddish-grey. The prevalent *Tattva* injects its particular hue. When by any act of ours one or more of these *Tattvas* is abnormally stimulated — as in states of excitement, anger, hatred, jealousy, or depression and manifold worries — it not merely upsets the balance of the prevalent *Tattvic* currents of the moment, but the disorder is stamped upon the current of the hour; and it passes on into the vast spaces of the Universe to return again and again with varying degrees of force according as the planets return to positions and relations one to another approximating the conditions at the time of the original disturbance.

All the misery in the world is primarily due to foul magnetisms (which are evil vibrations of tremendously penetrative and compelling power) generated by wrong and impure thoughts and by fear, and constantly fed by the crimes of the depraved and the sins of the weak. The world has grown old trying to punish crime out of existence. But it can never be lessened till the leaven of spiritual thought reaches the masses; and the basic truth, that wholesome, joyful thinking makes healthy, happy people is universally *known*.

It is possible to gain such power over the *Prânic* currents through perfect concentration — right thinking held steadfastly to the desired end — and careful attention to breathing correctly and rhythmically, as to put them in any *Tattvic* state desired; and this frees one from all antagonistic influences, whether hereditary or the chance (?) of birth — that is, planetary conditions at the moment. "Neither the lunar day, nor the constellations, nor the solar day, nor planet, nor god [that is, force]" have power to affect one who knows the *Tattvic* Law and applies it through habitual practice and right direction of thought and willpower. A human soul is more to God than any planet, and all the creative powers of the Universe work with and for the right.

Throughout the Universe we have the seven-fold division, and that the planets are closely related with this, having each a correspondence with plane and principle and element, with color and with tone, is so manifest to the Occult student as to need no demonstration. We are so wonted to this seven-fold division in some of the common affairs of life as to accept it unquestioningly. Thus, the seven days of the week are named from the planets, not in haphazard fashion, but strictly in accordance with their movements hour by hour.

A cardinal tenet of the earliest known principles of astrology was that every hour and every day is under the direct rule and influence of a planet; and there is no record of a period when the nearer planets, from Saturn to Mercury, were not known and symbolized as in our era. Of these, the sun and moon, supposed by the Egyptians to circle round the earth, were recognized as paramount in influence upon it; and the others were dignified according to the periods of their orbits which were the gauge of their distance.

The planet ruling the first hour names the day, and the succession begins with Saturn, the most distant, and takes the planets in their order, viz.: Saturn, Jupiter, Mars, Sol, Venus, Mercury, and Luna. Thus, on Saturn's day Jupiter rules the second hour; Mars, the third; Sol (sun), the fourth; Venus, the fifth; Mercury, the sixth; and Luna, the seventh. Every planet reigns the first hour of its own day, and the eighth, fifteenth, and twenty-second. Three repetitions carry us through the twenty-first hour; Saturn rules the twenty-second; Jupiter, the twenty-third; and Mars the twenty-fourth, finishing the day. Then Sol rules the first hour of the succeeding day, which is Sunday; called by the Romans *Dies Dominica,* or Lord's Day,— the day of the Lord Sun. Some authorities count from the rising of the sun; but a very old work, *Arcandum's Astrology,* reckons this planetary rule of hours *from midnight* which agrees with the modern reckoning of time.

The orderly repetition brings Luna — the moon — in as ruler of the next day, hence, Monday; Mars, (French, *Mardi*), Tuesday; Mercury, Wednesday; Jupiter, (Saxon, Thor), Thursday; and Venus (Saxon, Frea), Friday. All of the Latin tongues preserve in the names for the days of the week their planetary origin; but the Saxon derivation of English nomenclature has in ours obscured it in part.

All possibility that chance or pure arbitrary selection had any part in thus naming the days seems eliminated when we consider the double harmony ruling the order. The succession of the planets is not only from the slowest, Saturn, to the swiftest, the moon; but also in the exact order of their distance from the earth, from the most remote to the nearest. In matters astrological it is this regular succession of the planets, hour by hour, that determines fortunate planetary hours for various acts and undertakings. They are not, however, the same for all persons, being modified in effect by the characteristics established at the nativity.

It is interesting while on the subject, and piles up the authority for thus naming the days of the week and their order as we know them, to mention that the seven Hebrew words for the first seven cardinal numbers are all formed of one syllable that signifies a star (or fire or light) and another expressing its quality, and they follow strictly the above order, beginning with Sunday as the first day of the week. This is conclusive evidence that at the earliest formation of that language the relation between the planets and the days of the week was recognized as a basic fact in nature. The characteristic influences of the several planets thus expressed in the Hebrew names agree perfectly with the attributes still commonly assigned them; and as they are important in our further study I give them here with the original uncorrupted form of the Hebrew numbers:

1. *Ash-shèd;* Sol, all-bountiful fire.
2. *Ash-nem;* Luna, star of slumber, star of oracles.

3. *Ash-lesh;* Mars, star of flame.
4. *Ar-rabo;* Mercury, star of activity.
5. *Chem-ash;* Jupiter, star of warmth, star of joy.
6. *Ash-ish;* Venus, star of existence.
7. *Ash-shebo;* Saturn, star of old age, and signifying also *the end and the beginning.*

In further consideration of planetary influences, there seem to be convincing reasons for observing scrupulously this natural order of the planets in time and space,— the only one which satisfies my mind as in harmony with the *Tattvic* Law. Confronted with the problem of harmonizing these, it was for a time bewildering to find how many tables of planetary correspondencies with color, number, metals, elements, and days had been devised in which the natural sequence of the planets is constantly violated, and the days of the week are thrown into utter confusion; Monday following Tuesday, and Saturday, Wednesday. There is but one solitary anchor of agreement upon these planetary correspondencies between the various tables, religious, Occult, astrological, and astronomical,— with but one exception, to my knowledge, all connect Mars with fire, heat and passion, and the strife that leads to armed contest; hence, he was called the god of war. We shall weigh the authority of some of these tables when we study in their turn color and number in greater detail.

Our immediate interest now is with the *Tattvic* correspondencies which subject their activities — that is, their vibrations — in physical organisms to planetary influences.

The *Shivâgama*, which is the Sanskrit authority for most of our knowledge concerning the *Tattvic* Law, gives two sets of *Tattvic* values or correspondencies for the planets, which at the outset is bewildering and unsatisfactory. There is but the slightest agreement between the two; and upon examination the logical mind rejects both as equally arbitrary and capricious, and seeks for a satisfactory hypothesis upon which to base the law of correspondencies.

We ask ourselves: How do the planets differ one from another in elementary substances, and how are the *Tattvas* differentiated? In the evolution of the latter (see Chapter V) we know that *Âkâsha* — the bowl in which all are mixed — is the most sublimated and that they increase in density as they descend to *Prithivi*, the activities of which tend to cohesiveness and compactness. This brings us immediately to the question: Are not the planets differentiated in the same way, and is not their density determined in like manner, or by the variation in the proportions of the *Tattvas?* If so, which is the most ethereal?

Fortunately modern science has arrived at very definite conclusions upon this subject of the density of the planets,— a triumph of mathematics, that wonderful science on the wings of which the most severely materialistic mind fares forth into the invisible and brings back irrefutable data. When we group the planets in the astronomical order of their density; we find that it increases in an almost regular progression from Saturn to Mercury, which harmonizes perfectly in sequence with the age-honored order of the hour-by-hour rule; that is, from the most distant to the nearest. The remote planets Uranus (Herschel) and Neptune (pronounced by Occultists to be outside our system) do not come within the relations we are considering. They were unknown and *invisible* to the ancient world. Both discovered within the last century and a quarter (1781-1846, respectively), their influence upon earth life as yet is very slight, but they are heralds of coming changes.

Dropping out of this planetary sequence, temporarily, during our search for *Tattvic* correspondencies, the sun and moon, lords respectively of the positive and negative currents of *Prâna*, we are reminded that the earth upon which we live is also a planet and has its place in this progression of density; and we find it between Venus and Mercury. But in her orbital distance from the sun, the earth's place in the sequence is between Venus and Mars. Remember this, for it will be found to explain a seeming *Tattvic* irregularity.

I do not expect those readers who have merely read these lessons so far, and have neither practiced nor studied, therefore do not know one *Tattva* from another nor recall their distinguishing characteristics, to grasp the significance of the above established facts. It is not mere phenomena we are seeking but absolute truth. And those who are beginning to know the separate *Tattvas* by their fixed activities and relations and invariable effects must already understand their logical correspondencies with the planets. Here is the opportunity to do some serious thinking. All interested students should meditate upon the subject and see how near they can come to a correct solution of the problem before reading the next chapter.

It is necessary to give extreme emphasis to the fact that these lessons are neither mere speculations nor simply disclosures of curious mysteries. They are the first attempt to explain, in so practical a manner as to apply to every human need, the basic truths, as far as human intelligence has yet unravelled them, concerning the vital force in human organisms. And their value is that they teach a thoroughly scientific method of personal training to obtain control of body and mind, and make them the perfect vehicles for the soul's expression that the Creator intended. Only by means of constant and regular practice of the breathing exercises and of concentration can these benefits be gained. In concentration the mind is gradually attuned to those Kosmic influences which in their very nature are antagonistic to the evil material inclinations that are hazards to physical health and check our evolutionary progress.

It is through the ability to control *Prâna* and center it wherever we desire that we build the ladder to perfect centralization; a state of pure concentration which is lofty aspiration and, releasing the soul from its physical chains, places it upon its own throne, and discloses to it the realms of knowledge and power to which it has access.

CHAPTER XV

THE ACTIVITIES OF THE MACROCOSM IN THE MICROCOSM

THE new science declares confidently that we are akin to the stars, meaning thereby that, being composed of like elements though in vastly different states, we have through countless ages evolved therefrom. Yet it would cut us off entirely from that influence now! And this is the great stumbling block of progress.

When science goes further and recognizes that mankind, as also every living creature and every visible, material thing, is ever in the making and has never been severed from that original kinship, humanity will gain an immense impetus in the upward ascent of the evolutionary spiral, towards the development of spiritual senses. The X-ray foreshadows the powers humanity will thus gain.

Fortunately, recent discoveries are fast undermining the walls between the visible and invisible that materialism has with such blind zeal endeavored to render impregnable. It is of vast significance to have discovered that "The chemistry of all parts of space is the same." The factor which they leave out of all their calculations and investigations is "The Life-Movement of the Spirit through the Rhythm of Things." This is the energy within energy behind all phenomena, the Soul of every atom, an energy of which we are a part, and of which we use whatever we will; that is, whatever we fit ourselves for through training of will and desire and thought.

Of stupendous import to the race is it to study present stellar influences, realizing that the most distant star that lights the midnight canopy has its not insignificant part to play in the Kosmic whole — just as every atom and molecule in the physical body has its use and connection with that whole. All phenomena, atmospheric, terrene, physical, or mental, may be traced to Kosmic energies, *a part of which we are.*

Every point in the macrocosm is a center of action and reaction for the whole ocean of *Prâna;* and every one of these centers has its own atmosphere with its special limit. Râma Prasâd says they might be called "solar atoms." They are "of various classes according to the prevalence of one or more of the constituent *Tattvas.*" And yet further, "Every atom has, therefore, for its constituents, all the four *Tattvas,* in varying proportions according to its position in respect of others. The different classes of these solar atoms appear on the terrestrial plane as the various elements of chemistry." These points — the most infinitesimal units of *time* as of *space* — are called *Trutis* in Sanskrit, and lacking a word to so clearly identify the thing, I shall use it. To understand the ceaseless play of vibratory rays emanating from the celestial workshops, meeting and crossing or impinging upon one another on varying planes, imagine, if you can, the spectacle presented if seven or more particles of radium could be so placed and displayed in a darkened room that you could see the criss-crossing of their brilliant rays in a bewildering maze.

At every intersection of rays there would be a *Truti* receiving those rays, but no two *Trutis* could possibly receive precisely the same vibrations, for not only are there three kinds of rays to move at varying tangents but the *Trutis* would vary in plane and also in distance from the centers. Just such streams of influence are beating upon us all the time. In the zone of earth-life, every *Truti* of the ecliptical space is an individual organism whose life-phases change with the momentary variations of the *Tattvic* vibrations as the earth and her sister planets whirl in their orbits.

Man is a microcosmic sphere of energy exactly duplicating or reflecting the macrocosmic sphere, of which he is as it were a single cell, made up of millions of atoms held together by vibratory law. Just as no two *Trutis* can be exactly alike, so no two human beings are, for the unceasing play of the *Tattvas* is a constant mingling and changing under the ebb and flow of the Great Breath, which holds all the planets and constellations in their assigned orbits. Thus the *Tattvas* are the forces that lie at the root of all manifestations. They are that which lies behind every natural phenomenon. But it is only when the *Tattvas* reach a certain state of density that they become visible. The sun, stars, and planets are the visible, materialized centers of invisible, spiritual and ethereal forces. To spiritual vision no matter is dense.

It should be remembered that no two planets move with the same velocity or in the same orbit, and that consequently their aspects one to another are incessantly changing. The varying forms of *Tattvic* force and influence cause this and it is the reaction from the planets which injects such variation in the *Prânic* currents flowing earthward; and, in consequence, into every species of earth organism — these organisms being, as you will remember, manifestations on the gross (that is, *visible!*) plane of *Tattvic* activities.

Astronomers have recognized that the mutual interaction between the planets is a never-ending source of perturbations and disturbances, now checking and diverting, now restraining and now accelerating each and every one in its orbit, so that their paths through the congeries of stars which form the constellations, though never diverging far from the ecliptic, are most devious, being marked by eccentric loops and kinks recoiling upon their celestial pathways. Size and weight or velocity of motion, and especially their position in relation to the sun have been the factors supposed to account for the influences and antagonisms driving these stellar lords to so erratic conduct.

That the antagonism was in substance, a question of chemical affinity or repulsion — shall we not say of electrical condition? — seems never to have occurred to investigators. But when we apply the *Tattvic* Law to the problem there is the most logical basis to believe that it solves the enigma, accounting for all vagaries and idiosyncrasies and for the known influences of one planet upon another.

Let us begin with Saturn. By our law of correspondencies, it seems a simple matter to recognize that this most masterful and significant of the major planets is the center of *Âkâshic* influence, and derives from the predominance of this *Tattva* all the malefic influences which the astrologer attributes to the " great infortune." The rays of light thus thrown upon the subject dissipate a cloud of mystery and make clear hitherto unexplainable phenomena, as also many a legend and story of old. Both Saturn and Jupiter are said to present " only a surface of clouds, and may not have anything solid about them;" but it is suspected that they have a high temperature. Some states of *Âkâsha* are known to be marked by an extraordinarily high temperature, and "a surface of cloud" is what we should naturally expect.

Even to the naked eye Saturn gleams with a cold blue light. Seen through a five-inch telescope, the planet appears of a cool silver-white color, with delicate greyish shadings, blending one with another as they stretch from the bright equatorial belt to the deep blue poles. These polar caps are sometimes described as of a dark greenish hue, but the great dissimilarity in human optics would account for this discrepancy, as also would changing *Tattvic* conditions. An interesting feature is that the planet is banded by vari-colored belts, red, orange, and sometimes delicate rose-color; they are, however, less brilliant than Jupiter's belts and not recognized as so variable.

But the greatest distinction of Saturn — the phenomenon that puzzles the scientists the most — is its remarkable system of rings, separate from the planet and surrounding its equatorial belt. There are two broad, bright bands, separated from each other by "a black line" (indigo?), which "line" marks a 1,600-mile gap; and a third dusky inner ring which is only faintly luminous and so transparent that the edge of the planet can be seen through its mass. The space between them has been measured and it is estimated to be from nine to ten thousand miles broad. The inner and outer rings are over 10,000 miles in width, and the middle one is more than a third broader, being 16,500 miles wide.

To the knower of the *Tattvas*, the only possible hypothesis is that these rings are *Tattvic* emanations from the mother bowl of *Âkâsha*, and their peculiarities so far as known perfectly agree with their natural identification. Thus, the "gauzy," "crepy" inner ring is *Vâyu* (air), whence emerges the brightest and broadest ring, *Tejas*. The expansive nature of this *Tattva* explains its greater width, and the qualities of light and heat and its characteristic color, its superior brilliancy. The outer ring appears to be *Prithivi*. Color and volume corroborate this suggestion, while in the midnight-gap that separates it from *Tejas*, *Âkâsha* must hold *Âpas* (water) in a latent state. This order of visibility corresponds perfectly with the planetary sequence, and also with the changes of the Tattvas in the currents of *Prâna* within our bodies, as described in Chapter XIII, where your attention was attracted to the peculiarity that the order of evolution (see Chapter V) was violated. I am satisfied that we find in the planetary sequence the explanation for this, and the famous rings of

Saturn corroborate the belief. No other planets have rings. Only from *Âkâsha* could they emanate.

Saturn's rings are the girdle with which Satan alone among the gods is girt about; for Satan is the Soul and spiritual ruler of Saturn. His kingdom is the house of matter. "Evil is the result of limitation, and Satan is the Lord of Limit" (see "Perfect Way," page 369). Remember that through *Âkâsha* spirit descended into matter.

Ancient myths represent Saturn as devouring his children, which symbolizes exactly what the *Âkâshic Tattva* does with every other *Tattva*. Ages before Christ, all the lesser celestial bodies were regarded as Saturn's children. The Hebrews had several names for Saturn, but as Sater, or Scater, the attributes conferred upon him will be recognized as symbolizing perfectly the qualities or powers of *Âkâsha*. He was called the "god of secrecy," "parent of successive being," and "author of generation." It was believed that Sater *consumed all things* and *again repaired them*. Men were in closer touch in those days with matters celestial to have felt the mysterious influences of all these things which it is our privilege to understand rationally as inherent in the power of one of the centers from which the life we live is flowing constantly to us.

Saturn's influence tends to fix more deeply that

of other planets. He rules the East wind which, moving contrary to the earth's motion, conduces greatly to dampness and depletes the electricity in the atmosphere. This is one reason why the East wind " gets onto " people's nerves. They are failing to receive the normal supply, but *the remedy is to generate it within.* Fear has always been recognized as the active expression of the Saturn principle, and certainly nothing more is needed to identify the *Akâsha* influence.

Now the soul and life of the whole Solar System is the solar orb, and the human " soul is as a spiritual sun, corresponding in all things with the solar orb." If it permits evil to exist in its sphere — the microcosm — that evil will attract corresponding astral influences from the macrocosm. Disturbing influences can thus, of course, enter the body as the *Tattvas* change in their normal course; but thought has the power either to subdue them when they appear or to repel them before they find entrance, through holding tenaciously thoughts of serene confidence. Imagination is the architect, and thought the builder. We must have a perfect plan and use good materials if we would protect our bodies from the external disturbing thought-influences to which every organ is more or less sensitive. Its *receptivity depends upon us.*

Excessive indulgence in the gratification of any special sense-pleasure tends to exaggerate the

Tattva ruling that sense to an unwholesome degree. Thus the intensifying of one color may be the *extinction* of others, and at least casts an evil shade upon them; and this, of course, affects the whole current of *Prâna,* disturbing the *Tattvic* balance. Many diseases, petty and grave, result from no other cause.

The fact must never be lost sight of that spiritual energy differs from physical energy almost as much as does light from darkness. It is not dependent upon these celestial currents of ether which carry the renewing elements of physical matter, but is itself one with that even more subtle force that permits them to manifest on the gross, visible plane. It is the only unchangeable Principle within us, the real substance which never disintegrates.

The power to control the physical self and make of it the perfect vehicle it is intended to be for the growth and development of this spiritual self, is gained more rapidly by persistent and regular practice of the Alternate and Held-breath exercises, and by thoughtful attention from time to time to deep rhythmic breathing, than by any other system of discipline and study or therapeutic régime that I know of. I have already advocated this so earnestly and so repeatedly that further word or explanation seems superfluous.

Exhaustion is due entirely to the disordered state of the human battery, and in this condition all organic functions are lowered in tone and quickly reflect that disorder. Neither lungs, skin, nor kidneys have sufficient energy to eliminate the rapidly accumulating wastes; hence vital centers become clogged, and serious disease sets in wherever the physical structure is weakest. The first need at such times is to renew the battery and restore the balance of the disordered currents of vital force; and the media for doing this — breathing exercises — is so simple, so easy to apply, that the most helpless invalid, if the mind be sane and capable of directing, can employ it for regenerating the whole being. Both nerve and blood circulation — and thereby *all functions* — are stimulated more by this method than by any possible physical culture exercises.

And here a caution is timely: There is a vast difference in attempting to exercise "healing" power from without, as when denying disease and pain, and working from within outward in affirmation of the desired condition. The resulting atomic vibrations and the potencies involved are very different. The one is a species of constraint, the other is free, upward guidance.

We must strive for poise and tranquillity, for repose and confidence; which, manifesting themselves in good colors — favorable *Tattvas* — draw good and pure colors, and help to build purer and stronger the life thus aiming for the highest and the best.

CHAPTER XVI

MORE ABOUT MACROCOSMIC ACTIVITIES IN THE MICROCOSM

WITH the identification of Saturn as the highest manifestation upon a visible plane of *Âkâshic* activity, the way is made plain for us to read God's handwriting in the heavens, where he plainly discloses the whole scheme of creation — the descent of spirit into matter through the gradually increasing density of the same, *primarily simple*, elements ever growing more complicated by repeated permutations as they become more gross.

This is the secret of the fact that "The chemistry of all parts of space is the same." But the puzzle of the scientist in all his investigations is the ever-recurring *Âkâsha* — the neutral point, the *Sushumnâ*, into which all activities disappear or merge. He calls it usually X; that is unknown — hence the X-ray; and the Gamma-ray of radium is thus classed. The ether of science is the grossest manifestation of *Âkâsha*, though Mme. Blavatsky says that on our plane, for us mortals, it is the seventh Principle of the astral light, and three degrees higher than radiant matter.

In Jupiter the predominant *Tattva* is *Vâyu*, next in order to *Âkâsha*. When near together Jupiter and Saturn disturb each other more than do any other planets. As there must be a close affinity between ether and air this is exactly what we should expect; but were it not for the vast space separating Jupiter from Mars — double the ratio of that between other planets according to Bode's symmetrical law of progression — there would be even greater disturbances when these two planets approach each other. As it is, the violent impact of their predominant *Tattvas* — Air and Fire — is the cause of thunder. The severity and prevalence of thunder storms depends upon their aspects one to another.

Examined through a large telescope, the *Tattvic* activities in Jupiter's globe present a beautiful picture of varied and changing color, olive-greens and purple mingling with the more predominant brown, red, and yellow. Although well-defined zones of reddish clouds — *Tejas* vibrations — stretch around the sphere parallel with Jupiter's equator, all these masses display the peculiarities of clouds, as in our earth atmosphere of air, moving with varying velocity in strong aerial currents and constantly changing their relative positions.

The equatorial belt itself, brilliantly lemon-hued or sometimes ruddy, shows *Prithivi*, and the region is sprinkled over with balloon-shaped white masses which are naturally *Âpas*. These move faster than the dark and brighter-hued masses. The famous " great red spot," of vast dimensions, is an exception to the other evanescent phenomena; for, though changing hue from time to time, its stability of position has been an important aid to the astronomer in ascertaining not merely data concerning Jupiter but important facts in physics. The rapidity of changes upon the surface of the planet indicate to the scientist " a temperature not much short of incandescence." We who know the qualities of the *Tattvas* can recognize the source of this as the *Tejas* of the " great red spot," the next *Tattva evolved after Vâyu*. Towards the poles of the planet the pure Jupiter vibration — *Vâyu* — is seen in a vast expanse of blue and blue-grey.

When favorably placed in a nativity, the influence of Jupiter promotes a fortunate and honored life, and therefore he has been called " the god of fortune." Seen with the naked eye the planet is a beautiful object, shining with a silvery-white light; and it was so placed during the winter of 1906-7 that no cloudless nights could possibly be very dark. On moonless nights Jupiter may cast a shadow on the snow.

Astrologically considered, Jupiter represents the

temperate, moist element in nature, its special function being to disintegrate and help to germinate; that is, to promote *change* in all things visible, and this we know to be the special attribute of *Vâyu*,— motion, tireless, ceaseless motion, for which *Âkâsha* is ever at hand providing the space. The color and number of Jupiter's *four* moons is further corroboration of the *Tattvic* Law. There are two blue satellites and one red and one yellow. The *Âpas Tattva* in the Jupiter atmosphere would reflect blue just as a body of water on the earth reflects the blue of an azure sky above it. Thus the Jupiter system reflects the law of system within system, every *Truti* of which manifests the whole law.

The characteristics of Mars, in which *Tejas* predominates, have always been so striking that there is a gratifying agreement in all speculations, records, and legends concerning the planet. There is great antagonism between Mars and Venus, as why should there not be since water extinguishes fire? Therefore, to secure a measure of stability, our earth comes between these natural enemies as a pacificator; and this greater planetary stability is reflected in the *Tattvic* changes in our bodies, which are smoother, more harmonious and imperceptible, flowing from *Tejas* into *Prithivi* and then into *Âpas* than could be the case if *Âpas* came next to *Tejas*.

Fevers and chills, blushing, and sudden waves of upheaving discord flowing through the body are all manifestations of disorder in the flow of the *Tattvas,* but more especially of *Tejas.* And always the remedy is to face the situation — no matter what the cause — with mental poise and confidence; directing, as long as the disturbance lasts, frequent repetitions of the exercise in Alternate Breathing, and regularly inhaling deep, full, rhythmic breaths. Remember that for all chilly conditions the Held Breath is most efficacious. It may be repeated, with concentration mainly upon the feet and the solar plexus, till perspiration is induced.

Through a telescope, Mars displays white at the polar caps; but the ardent, fiery orb appears, even to the naked eye when favorably situated for observation, of a reddish or orange hue. The fiery strength of *Tejas* vibrations, called into increased activity by all emotion and by intense feeling and by love, have always been recognized as stimulating the passions of man to strife and war; hence Mars was the god of war. During the rare periods of peace in Old Rome, all the panoply and pageantry of war, including the gorgeous red mantles, were treasured in the Temple of Mars.

The planet Mars is said to be always an enemy of Mercury, but this is the evil aspect of Mars— the contentious state of the planetary vibrations which struggle against the higher and purer conditions of the Mercury influence. These are felt by all human beings in the proportion that they permit themselves to be swayed by passion and excitement without restraint of reason and will. Even so-called "just" indignation injects disorder disturbing the rhythm and harmony of *Tattvic* activities within, and should be shunned.

When fortunately placed at birth the influence of Mars gives to a character earnestness, patience, determination, and courage combined with gentleness. But the cruel, tyrannical, unjust man, always quarrelsome and often a vain boaster, is under the influence of Mars' most malefic vibrations. He is his own worst enemy, but unfortunately makes an atmosphere of unhappiness wherever he may be. He can win his freedom only through self-conquest, and that is what his free will is for. I must insistently reiterate that every human being has the power to choose between the *Tattvic* vibrations which may thrill him with harmony or rend him with discord. The rays of certain *Tattvic* states will be reflected only when the surface is akin. Our thoughts govern that and attract to us our affinities. If we think passion and hate, *Tejas* is ever ready to supply the fuel. Every exhibition of ungoverned passion in man is a microcosmic cyclone, the path of whose

More About Macrocosmic Activities 179

destruction is limited only by the chances of environment.

Although the earth, the most important planet to us, is commonly ignored in considering the planetary correspondences with the *Tattvas*, and the source of the *Prithivic* current has been severally attributed to the Sun, Mercury, and Jupiter, I deem this not merely short-sighted but a grave error, the only rational solution of which is that it was done in the first place " as a blind "— a reason Mme. Blavatsky assigns for many puzzles. To do this is to take the earth out of its orbit, so to speak, and make of it an exception to the law. It is but logical to believe that as the *Âkâshic* current emanates in greater force from Saturn, and the *Vâyu* from Jupiter, so does also the *Prithivic* current emanate as the ruling *Tattva* from our Mother Earth. If we accept this as proved through the invariability of Natural Law, it explains perfectly the reason for the preponderating flow of *Prithivi* in our *Prânic* life-currents (see Chapter XIII). It is the *Tattva* of our environment, and in its normal flow puts us and holds us in sympathy with that environment.

Now, please do not ask me how you are to know when this *Tattva*, or any other special one, is flowing normally or is disturbed. I have described the varied activities and effects of the different *Tattvas* within the human entity with much more detail than has ever been before attempted. I have analyzed them as only long study and unceasing practice and experiment could enable one to do, and I gladly give to you the benefit of my research expressed as fully and as clearly as love for the task and enthusiasm of purpose can do it. I cannot, however, supply the application and the perseverance *individually needed* before *you can make this detail your own*. Without the exercise of these faculties, you can never hope to gain a practical knowledge of the *Tattvas*. It is not a thing that can be poured over you " in words, mere words." *You must think yourself.* Remember what I told you in an early chapter: that the Hindu teacher never imparts any fact to a student which by *long meditation* he can find out for himself.

It is not by once reading, but only after many readings and *much thinking* that you can reasonably expect to master the mass of detail contained in these chapters; the difficulty being the greater because the subject is — to most readers — absolutely novel. But it is only by thus mastering it that anyone can make a personal application of this Law of Life.

When our feet press the earth we receive the strongest and purest vibrations of *Prithivi*, which is the secret of the exhilaration we feel when we can get into the real country, and of the benefit to nerves and soul derived from long country tramps. This fact also discloses the deep philosophy of Father Kneipp's barefoot treatment. In the early morning, before the day's struggle and conflict have generated discord (this especially in large communities where human beings are herded closely), the vibrations are at the highest state of harmonic activity; and when the feet tread the dew-wet grass, the double benefit is gained of receiving the two most favorable *Tattvas* in their freshest and most refined, highly electrified states. On our planet, the *Prithivi* vibrations are negative to *Tejas* (Mars) and positive to *Âpas* (Venus); thus water is negative to the earth. Most dwellers in large cities, where the earth is for the most part solidly incased in stone and brick and asphalt, are grievously handicapped, for it is seldom that their feet come in direct contact with Mother Earth. The efficacy of mud-baths is derived from the earth vibrations, but like benefits can be obtained by encouraging in more congenial ways the flow of *Prithivi!*

The planetary influence of Venus upon terrestrial life is very important as the *Âpas Tattva* which predominates in that near and brilliant planet is the unifying element that gives to organized matter its quality of stability. In dry seasons all the green things of earth suffer and many of them quickly fade and perish because Mars unites with the Sun to divert or absorb the cooling and refreshing *Âpas* vibrations from Venus, and their own rays increase proportionally in fervor and burning power.

As five-sixths of the human body is composed of water it is of the utmost importance that opportunity be given for the fullest normal play of the *Âpas Tattva;* and this, you will remember, requires that the lowest cells in the lungs be filled. Tight-lacing inhibits this absolutely, as it holds the lower lobes of the lungs in a vise-like grip; and usually it prevents anything approaching a free movement of the diaphragm. The practice is slow suicide, yet women revive the iniquitous custom — as at present — whenever fashion gives the command. The stability of *Âpas* is recognized in that manifestation of *Prâna* which is known as *Vyâna;* the force which, during life, keeps the whole body in shape and resists the breaking down and disintegration of its tissues.

Next to the deprivation of fresh air, perhaps the most prolific source of human ills is from stinting the body in its supply of pure water inside and out. As a rule, those who drink water most freely, take it when they should not,— with their meals, when the important digestive fluids need to be undiluted in order to put in their fine work. The greatest benefit derived from visits to famous European "cures" is due not half so much to the special virtue of the mineral water as to the fact that for several weeks the business of life is the drinking of water in quantities limited only by the ability to swallow it. If people formed the habit of drinking pure water freely between meals and, especially, the last thing at night and the first thing in the morning, they would not need to " take the cure."

Water is the mystical symbol of the soul because it is ever chemically pure. While it is the great solvent, it is also the absolvent and purifier, for whatever of foulness it takes up is held in suspension and can be eliminated by distillation. And thus it is with the soul. Its " saving " is the choice of freeing itself from the passions and errors of the material, sense life. The pure, self-controlled soul and the physical body wherein it dwells — which ever and always reflects the power controlling it — are alike freed from the Karma and the impurity of unfavorable planetary vibrations which sow discord and incite to evil.

Never lose sight of the fact that the Sun is the source of the *Prânic,* or life-current, which contains in itself all the *Tattvas;* but the variations in the proportions of the *Tattvas* injected into the life-current come from the planetary currents, in every one of which the ruling *Tattva* of the planet predominates. It is interesting to know that the spectrum of Venus shows the presence of watery vapor.

Thus it is that the activities of the macrocosm are reflected in the microcosm.

It is in the pulmonary manifestation of *Prâna* that the *Tattvic* condition of the vital currents can be most indisputably ascertained; for every *Tattva* throws the elastic spongy cells of the lungs into the from of its characteristic vibration. Thus when the *Âpas Tattva* is prevalent, the cells expand in crescent-like shape. When *Tejas* predominates, they are triangular, and with *Vâyu*, spherical; and various modifications of these geometrical forms indicate the *Tattvic* permutations. The test suggested for examining these is to hold a brilliant-surfaced mirror before the mouth to intercept the exhalations. The vapor as it condenses upon the cool surface will take the form of the vibration dominant at the moment; and it can be best seen by another person looking over the shoulder of the one whose breath is under examination, as of course these vapor cells are extremely evanescent.

We have now identified the planetary correspondencies with all the *Tattvas*, and there yet remains the smallest and swiftest of the heavenly host, Mercury, who yields nothing in importance to the more brilliant and better-known orbs. He is the bond of union, and truly "the messenger of the gods." How he performs this office I shall try to make plain in the next chapter.

CHAPTER XVII

MERCURY AND THE ACTIVITIES OF THE SUSHUMNÂ

"HERMES, as the messenger of God, reveals to us His paternal will, and — developing in us intuition — imparts to us knowledge. The knowledge which descends into the soul from above, excels any that can be attained by the mere exercise of the intellect."

This quotation from the Neoplatonist Proclus is a most fitting introduction to our study of the influence of the planet Mercury — called by the Greeks, "Hermes"— upon human life, for by the illuminating light of the *Tattvic* Law we are able to remove the statement from the realm of " mere speculation," to which it has been indulgently relegated for centuries, and to feel convinced of the intuitional truth embodied in the ancient Greek thought. All scientific data concerning the planet Mercury as well as the fables and ancient myths connecting planet and god are strictly in harmony with what I believe to be Mercury's activities and influences, whether heavenly or terrestrial.

Briefly reviewing the first mentioned, we learn that as a stellar body Mercury is exceptional in many ways, and has always baffled the astronomer in his efforts to obtain accurate data concerning its constitution and environment. It is the smallest planet in diameter but the swiftest in motion; has the least mass but the greatest density, being two and one-fourth times denser than the earth, and only slightly less dense than the metal mercury; is nearest to the sun and has the most eccentric orbit. As seen from the sun, Mercury passes through one constellation of the Zodiac in a fraction over seven days, completing the circuit of the Zodiac in eighty-eight days; and as seen from the earth it makes three complete circuits of the sun in three hundred and forty-eight days. Also from our point of view, the planet is usually in the same constellation with the sun, and is never farther away than a nearby sign.

The astronomer considers it more than doubtful if Mercury has any atmosphere, and it has no satellite. When it can be observed in the same telescopic field with Venus, its totally different constitution is plainly betrayed by its markedly lower *Albedo*, or reflecting power; for Mercury appears as zinc or lead contrasted with the dazzling silver-white radiance of Venus. Now, I should like you to remember, in this connection, that wherever or whenever the *Âpas Tattva* — most prevalent in Venus — can be isolated, it is recognized by its glistening silvery whiteness. It is said to impart a silvery edge to the human aura.

I wish I knew how many of my readers could answer the question: What are the three principal *Nâdis* in the physical body? Those who cannot would better re-read Chapter XII. and fix firmly in their minds the names and offices of " the great main reservoir and conduits of life-force." You will understand perfectly then that the *Pingalâ*, on the right side of the spine, is the conduit of the solar current (positive), and the *Idâ*, on the left side, of the lunar current (negative); and, therefore, these *Nâdis* correspond respectively with the sun and the moon and are influenced by their activities. With what does the *Sushumnâ*, in which the two currents meet, correspond?

In our study of planetary relations and influences, we have traced the correspondence of the organic activities in the human body with the whole solar system, and the truth of the old Greek aphorism, " As it is above, so is it below," has been made to us a living reality. " When once your attention is drawn to the fact, you will constantly come upon proof that to many ancient people this was a familiar truth. Bacon says the ancients styled man, " a little world in himself." Now, the correspondence of the constellations of the Zodiac and the planets with all the organs of the human body through *its nervous system* is but the microcosmic reflection of the vast system of Kosmic vibrations. Therefore, in the solar system we must find the Kosmic *Sushumnâ* in which the solar and lunar currents meet.

In the progress of the human soul, in its evolution, its growth and development, there is nothing more important than the office of the *Sushumnâ*. Consequently it is inconceivable that it has not a Kosmic prototype of equal importance to the solar system. In the gloaming, at dawn and at twilight, the solar and lunar currents meet in the Kosmic *Sushumnâ*. The identification of Mercury as this *Sushumnâ* of the macrocosm makes perfectly clear and comprehensible all the dignities, attributes, and influences which legend and fable have conferred upon the planet, both actually and symbolically; and explains many of the characteristics that have puzzled the astronomer. No other planet possesses any attributes that connect it with the office of the *Sushumnâ*.

Again giving precedence to known facts, our first clue is that Mercury is in the closest Kosmical relation to the sun. Indeed, so close is it that only the patient observer who keeps in touch with the movements of the planet and knows when and where to look for it ever sees it. There is a tradition that the eyes of Copernicus were never gratified by the sight of this swift solar attendant. In the latitude of New York and neighboring States, for about a fortnight during its greatest Eastern elongation from the sun, Mercury can be seen in the early twilight just before its setting; and for a like period when the planet is West of the sun, rising before the orb of day, it can be seen in the early dawn. During the first weeks of December, 1906, Mercury was a morning star, and was seen in close companionship with Venus. These neighboring planets were in Scorpio; and only two signs to the Southwest, in Virgo, the crescent of the waning moon was in conjunction with Mars. The spectacle was unforgetably beautiful,— worth many early risings to enjoy.

It was a reminder, also, that both esoterically and astrologically, Mercury and Venus are considered spiritual affinities, while Mars and Saturn are thought to have a close physical sympathy. This latter may be beneficial or harmful according as the physical is kept under subjection and subordinated to its divinely planned office as a perfectly fitted vehicle for the soul's activities, or is given free rein and stifles all higher interests.

Now, Mercury is the unifying element between the several Principles of man as between the *Tattvas*. The strife the planet arouses is that it is ever impelling upward and resists downward tendencies. It is Mercury's rod that pricks the conscience and would ever extend its support in the struggle against wayward impulses. When you fully understand the entire office of the *Sushumnâ*, this will be quite plain.

Both the density and the swiftness of Mercury are accounted for, or explained, by the *Tattvic* state of *Prâna* when in the *Sushumnâ*. Of course it is the same in the macrocosm as in the microcosm, only on a vaster scale. Though apparently quiescent during the moment of conjunction, the quiescence is but seeming. The concentrated energy of the *Tattvas* through their closely compacted atoms in the united currents as they meet in the *Sushumnâ* produces a state of extreme density. During concentration, when alone the higher office of the *Sushumnâ* is called into activity, the velocity of the vibrations is stimulated to an inconceivable speed.

(Six months after this study of Mercury's influences was first set in type, I had the extreme gratification of finding the following corroboration of my belief. Alchemists knew " Mercury has to be ever *near Isis* [the moon] *as her minister*, as without Mercury neither Isis nor Osiris [the sun] can accomplish anything in their great work."—*Secret Doctrine*, Vol. 1, p. 388).

Curiously enough, we have in the rise of mercury in a thermometer a perfect symbol of the rise of the

Activities of the Sushumnâ

vital force in the *Sushumnâ*, for the state of increased activity and density and vastly increased velocity is also one of rising temperature. The spinal *Sushumnâ*, which we have now specially to consider, is a hollow canal in the center of the spinal cord. In ordinary persons who are absorbed in trivialities and purely material interests, it is closed at the base, the point of union between the *Pingalâ* and *Idâ*, where the residual nervous action — the memory of sensations — is stored in the sacral plexus. This canal is the so-called Occult channel of *Prâna*, through which, *when roused to activity*, the coiled-up latent *Prâna*, or *Kundalini*, ascends from the sacral plexus to the brain, and striking upon the pituitary body (the will-energizer) stimulates it to such activity that it in turn kindles the spiritual fire of the pineal gland. The first hint the student has that he is rousing this slumbering power is a sensation of warmth in the basic plexus — the *Mulâdhâri* of the Yogi — where it is "coiled-up"; and as the soul-governed will controls *Prâna* and holds it to the ascent through the canal, the heat increases.

All aspirations for higher things, all exaltation of prayer and worship, tend to set free a minute portion of this *Kundalini*, the "coiled-up one." Thus, you see, the path to "the Mystic Realm of the Undiscovered" leads through the *Sushumnâ*. We enter it in meditation. Often unknowingly, it is traversed by many a rapt enthusiast, and by the ardent inventor who wrests Nature's secrets from her vast repositories. Intuitional truths are never discovered elsewhere. Swâmî Vivekânanda says: " Wherever there is any manifestation of what is ordinarily called supernatural power or wisdom, there must have been a little current of *Kundalini* which found its way into the *Sushumnâ*."

The data concerning Mercury's close association with our spiritual natures is practically without limit, as he who begins to search will find. The symbol of the planet expresses the trinity or three in one, the circle representing the Spirit because without beginning or end. The crescent is the reflection, or Soul,— the negative of the Spirit as is the Moon of the Sun; and the cross typifies the four elements of the physical, or gross, plane of activity. There are four elemental divisions, called the " triplicities," of the Zodiac, and Mercury's influence in the varying signs is distinct. The astrologer Hazelrigg finds all the planetary symbols equally significant with that of Mercury, and believes none to be arbitrary signs, which is in agreement with all Occult teaching.

In all ancient lore, we find Mercury accredited as ruling the mind. Everywhere in myth and story he is sent as the interpreter and messenger to the *understanding* and *reason* of man. Even the thievish disposition attributed to Mercury symbolized the facility with which reason and understanding appropriate all knowledge. The very term *thought* is said by Anna Kingsford to be "the Egyptian equivalent for Hermes, the God Thaut, frequently written Thoth; these being for the Greeks and Egyptians the personification of the Divine Intelligence," that is, His messenger. The same Spirit was manifested to the Hebrew as Raphael,— like Hermes called "the physician of souls;" and to the Hindu as Buddhi.

One of the chief glories of Hermes was his conquest of the hundred-eyed Argus, which denotes, Mrs. Kingsford says: "The victory of the understanding over fate. For Argus represents the power of the stars over the unenfranchised soul." This corroborates what I have constantly endeavored to make emphatic, that the power of human thought guided by reason can change the planetary currents. The powers of reason and understanding to which Mercury guides us are above mere cold intellection. It is the stifling of pure reason by the exaltation of the human sense-governed mind that produced the rank materialism which has marked recent decades and from which Higher Thought is freeing the race of mankind.

The Roman name Mercury, by which we designate the planet, comes from *merx*, merchandise. Their god was of a much more material and sordid character than the Greek Hermes with whom they identified him, which betrays the truth that the people had degenerated and become more material. They chose to degrade "Hermes * * * Archangel, who bears the rod of knowledge by which all things in heaven and earth are measured" (*The Perfect Way*, p. 367), to a crafty, commercial god.

The farther back we go the more elemental, more spiritual are all the gods. Zeus is believed to have meant originally "the glistening ether." Hindu genius spiritualizes its sense-conceptions with wonderful readiness. The more remotely their myths are traced the more "atmospheric" do they become. The more the god merges with the planet and its ensouling Force.

A concluding word as to practice: When our wills hold our minds in check and thus restrain the scattering of forces through wasteful and, oftener than not, discordant activities, the *Prânic* currents flow rhythmically and gather force and strength as all the molecules of the body yield to the harmony and tend to *move in the same direction*,— which means a tremendous gain in electric power: Only by the uplift of this conscious direction can we connect with the great Central Dynamo, the Divine Spirit.

Thus the soul-directed thought is electrical, itself a ray of spiritual powers, the effectual energy of which is gauged by the steadfastness of purpose, the soul-force, which directs it. Never forget that the mind which is the disturber and disorganizer, creating all discord, when brought under control is the agent of our freedom. There is no limit to the power of thought.

CHAPTER XVIII

VITAL CENTERS FOR CONCENTRATION

IT should be very clear to my readers, now, that subtle bonds of rhythmic influence connect every human being with the vast spaces of the universe, and open to him illimitable resources if he but uses them aright. But alas! This is the *crux* of the problem. How many use them aright? Even the knowing how does not confer the power to do. Desire and will decide that! IT IS ONLY THROUGH USE THAT KNOWLEDGE BECOMES A HABIT AND THEN A POWER!

What is the purpose of concentration? It is to develop power; to develop the best there is in the individual through gaining control of the lower Principles and using the higher ones latent in every human being. But let me say at the outset of this study, lest some students have an entirely erroneous idea of our object: *It is not to develop psychic powers.* No; our object — a forecast of which was given in the last chapter — is far higher, vastly more important. It is, first, to complete the work which I trust is already well begun — the effort to obtain control of the mind; that wonderful instrument through which the dynamic power of thought manifests; by controlling which alone we can hope to *exercise the power for good only*.

Not till we quiet the mind's useless activities, and can hold it in leash, an obedient servant as it was designed to be, can we hope to attain the higher reward of concentration — the joy — the benediction — of a realization of soul-consciousness. This once achieved places a power for good under the control of a soul-directed Will that can never fail its possessor in any crisis.

A certain measure of development of the psychic senses comes as a natural attribute of growing spirituality, but this is not a real attainment in itself or *for itself;* and it varies greatly in degree in different constitutions and according to how it is employed. When made an end and aim by absorption in its phenomena, the activities of mere astral life which may be even more trivial than on this terrestrial plane, it leads to gross abuse of the powers; blocks irretrievably self-conquest and spiritual development, and invites untold misery in manifold forms.

You have learned that thought is the creator of force within these bodies; that is, the form of force active within is largely determined by the mind's habitual thoughts, and the ratio of the vibrations by the plane of its activity. Thus it is a demonstrable fact, a basic law of nature too long ignored, when not vehemently denied, that with every thought, since the mind reflects its vibrations upon the physical plane below, we are moulding these bodies of ours to ease or disease (see Chapter III). Then the greatest need of every human being is to gain control of the mind, and put a stop forever and aye to the discordant hash which the uncontrolled mind contrives to mix out of the ordinary events and duties of life from hour to hour.

Not until you can control your body *through you mind being brought under control,* will you be freed from that body's whimsies! When you have conquered the vehicle (the body), it will be your willing, skillful servant, fulfilling its divinely planned purpose of furthering growth and development instead of hampering it. Therefore, before progress can be made upon the spiritual plane, it is absolutely necessary to obtain physical and mental control, to bring the lower Principles into working harmony. When we know what the ideal is, as Swâmi Vivekânanda said: "What remains is to practice the methods of reaching it."

The Swâmi's inspired aphorisms prefatory to *Râja Yoga* are of deep significance here:

"EACH SOUL IS POTENTIALLY DIVINE. THE GOAL IS TO MANIFEST THIS DIVINITY WITHIN BY

CONTROLLING NATURE, EXTERNAL AND INTERNAL."

This mischievous mind, which uncontrolled turns many a paradise into purgatory, can be controlled for good only through a soul-directed and governed WILL, and nothing else so hastens the attainment of this mental control — the first stepping-stone towards the realization of soul-power — as the practice of Concentration. As you must well understand now, it is the only method of rousing the *Kundalini;* also called "The Tree of Knowledge," being the latent *Prâna,* or stored-up residual sensations in the great root-receptacle, or basic plexus. When this force, sleeping in every human being, is awakened through concentration it ascends the spinal canal by slow stages from one center to another, gathering strength in every *Padma,* till it rouses the potencies in the brain-centers of real illumination. This effort brings us under the most beneficent influence of Mercury,— an influence that is ever striving to purify us and lift us to higher planes of living and thinking.

Moreover, concentration is the only entrance to the blessed realm of Silence; that wordless space vibrant with peace; the peace of exquisitely subtle spiritual force, where we come in touch with the soul of things and thereby find our own souls. In the unspeakable peace of this precious Silence, the world of the senses disappears in a conscious rapport with the vaster universe of living thought which needs no words to clothe its meaning. It is the " Knowledge space " of the *Yogi*.

If you but think of it we are on the verge of Silence at every moment of existence. Its omnipresence laps us round about as the Universe of the invisible and inaudible, teeming with activities so infinitely finer, more subtle, that they escape cognizance by our grosser sense-perceptions. At any instant when we can shut out the consciousness of this physical environment we open the avenues of that consciousness to this inner silent world, and the importance of the experience is incalculable. Every time we attain it, the way is made easier to repeat the experience till it carries us to the full realization of the real subjective self.

Remember what I said in an early chapter: The life-current is more subtle than radio-activity, and it depends upon ourselves to how high power we shall raise it. The holding the attention — all our consciousness — to a given point, as when centering upon a special plexus or organ, accelerates the velocity of the *Tattvic* vibrations and, therefore, the force of *Prâna*. This effect and benefit are the immediate reward for the regular practice of the Held-Breath exercise for *Prânâyâma,* in which, through the polarization of the vital currents greatly increased power is generated and the

Vital Centers for Concentration 201

whole nervous system is energized. The benefit derived from the exercise is in exact ratio to the success of the student in holding the current mentally to the designated center. A good beginning is thus made in mental control, for the brain appropriates its full share of the energy, gains steadiness and flexibility, and the memory is quickened. All mental effort is made easier and more fruitful, and the voice — so intimately associated with our mentality — gains sweetness and fullness of tone, evidencing the increasing harmony of the life. All harsh, uneven, and strident tones can thus be overcome.

In concentration we develop still higher power — the power of higher forces on higher planes of activity. With regard to these varying planes, please remember that every one is positive to the next below and negative to the one above; and that the higher they are the finer, swifter, and more subtle are the vibrations. As you progress, gaining more and more control over the physical, and insight into the mental activities of your being, you will receive irrefutable proof that the spirit brings out power wherever it is focused.

When there is a state of physical discord and the need is to purify and harmonize the *Tattvic* vibrations on the physical plane as well as to obtain mental control, the most important centers upon which to concentrate are the sacral and the solar plexuses; the pituitary body (high up back of the throat), which is intimately connected with the ninth and tenth cranial nerves; and that core of the brain, the pineal gland.

The sacral plexus is so-called because situated in the sacrum; a composite bone formed of the union of the vertebrae between the lumbar and the coccygeal regions of the spine, containing the dorsal part of the pelvis. In man the sacrum, or sacred bone, is triangular, and consists of *five* vertebrae. This shape conforms to the basic plexus which it shelters, and proclaims it a dominating center of *Tejas* activity, whence this *Tattva's* stimulating vibrations speed to all the organs in this part of the body. No other *Tattva* responds so instantly to a thought, or to a glance from a speaking eye; for, remember, *Tejas* is regnant in the optic nerves. Therefore, as behind every thought is desire, the harmonious activity of *Tejas* in these vital organs depends upon the purity, saneness, and wholesomeness of our *desires;* and their control by a *soul-governed Will* affects the human life beyond all other influences. It is the difference between aspiring to be Godlike, and yielding to be the shuttlecock of the physical senses.

This is, of course, the turning point in life, for we all *are* and *become* what our *desires mould*. Desire prompts the Will to action. Shall it be a lawless ruler? Right here is the most prolific

Vital Centers for Concentration

source of evil. It is easier far to drift with desire; but know, once for all, it is the path of discord, the sower of disturbance.

In the Zodiac we find the clue to these close relations of organic sympathy which affect human life and character so profoundly. The constellation Scorpio is the symbol of desire because it exercises a paramount influence upon the physical center where desires are generated. This activity is assigned to the coccygeal gland (also known as Luschka's gland), situated near the extremity of the spinal column. This gland is most intimately associated with the arteries and nerves; but its exact function, like that of the spleen, pituitary body, and pineal gland, still remains a mystery to the anatomist. Scorpio is one of the "houses" of Mars. Now thought, under the influence of Sagittarius (next East of Scorpio as seen in the Heavens) is either above or below desire exactly according to the direction of our thoughts. If these are of the earth, earthy, the direction of these stellar influences is downward from Aries, governing the head, to Pisces ruling the feet.

The familiar figure of man in the almanacs shows the commonly assigned influence of the zodiacal signs upon different parts of the body. Familiar as it is, though, how little the illustration signifies to the majority of mankind! Yet the connection is deeply significant; and to a certain degree it is natural, normal, and healthful. You have learned that the soles of the feet are centers of *Prithivic* activity, and that in the contact of the feet with Mother Earth the flow of pure *Prithivi* vibrations is greatly stimulated. This *Tattvic* emanation received from the earth is an extremely subtle, ethereal magnetism which exhilarates the whole body. Whether the elemental forces which develop as this subtle *Tattva* ascends and stimulates and mingles with *Tejas* shall be purely physical or shall be transmuted into purer and higher principles depends upon its use or abuse.

The guide to both paths is in the Zodiac. For still within man is the Occult spiritual Zodiac which, corresponding exactly with that of the macrocosm, is circular. In this, notice particularly that Sagittarius is *above* Scorpio, and that Pisces — the abstract symbol of the will and influencing it — reflects its power upon desire in a vertical ray from above as in the physical Zodiac it reflects it from below. Accepting the guidance of Mercury and governing the body by reason and understanding we develop the power to employ all its mysterious forces for good. By controlling his desires through the power of thought — much easier than he who has never tried to dreams — man enters the upward, spiritual path, thus overcoming the downward and outward flow of his activities and emotions to things purely physical through the stimulus of his sense perceptions.

Notice also with care that it is not the will but thought which must first be employed to control desire and give it an upward impulse. Until this is accomplished, will is at the mercy of desire and but strengthens its evil intents. The moment thought, which directs and controls desire, recognizes its own agency, refuses to be swayed by impulses, and gains the mastery, the Will ascends to its higher plane, and its reflection transmutes desire to loftier aims; for Will and desire are the higher and lower aspects of one and the same thing. It is by the proper exercise of our Will that we accomplish all things on the higher planes and free our souls from physical chains.

Thus in all this overcoming we are building character, shaping destiny. And the petty trials, the small frictions of life are just as important if allowed to do their work of discord as seemingly more important matters. They demand their corresponding measures of resistance,— not the resistance of struggle, but the more effective resistance of poise, ensuring the calm spirit that commands reason and, therefore, can meet the annoyance with wise judgment.

Be not anxious if at first when trying to concentrate and enter the Silence a multitude of thoughts flit through the mind. It is the beginning of discipline to watch these vagaries. They will surprise you, but you will soon realize that you yourself are above and superior to the mind. You will separate yourself from it; and next will come the calm and confidence derived from consciousness of power to check and control the whole unruly tribe of trouble-makers and peace- and mind-destroyers. This, however, is not gained in a day, nor is it the reward of irregular, haphazard practice.

The influence of the Zodiac upon other vital centers, showing what is gained by concentration upon them, will be fully explained as we continue this study of the inter-relations of man and the Universe.

In all practice, assume an easy, erect posture (not "slumping" nor lounging; that is). This is especially important in the Held-Breath exercise; for as the object in view is to obtain control of *Prâna*, the region of the principle *Nâdis* through which the currents flow must be free from all constraint or strain. These lessons ought to have convinced everyone already that *at all times* any pressure upon the spinal column is an iniquitous menace to the very reservoir of life. But especially during periods of practice should attention be given to the absolute freedom of the spine and chest which should form an erect support for the neck and head poised in line above them. To twist or crook the spine during meditation or when concentrating the *Prāna* in different plexuses will not merely defeat the purpose but may cause disturbance, just as electric wires, if crossed and tangled, raise the mischief!

CHAPTER XIX

THE CONNECTION OF THE ZODIAC WITH VITAL CENTERS

YOU are now prepared to appreciate the significance of the statement that the constellations of the Zodiac severally reflect every stage of the involution of the Spirit into matter and its evolution out of it. Every zodiacal sign is the geometrical symbol of a great truth and fundamental law of existence; for it corresponds with successive stages in racial development through its connection with some physical center and the abstract principle which that center influences.

The internal man is formed in the image of the whole Kosmos, and the germ of correspondence with every principle, from the lowest to the highest, is in every human being. All aspiration and striving for excellence, all recognition of the value of the best, even on the material plane, and dissatisfaction with anything short of that best, is the struggle of these potentialities for recognition and for opportunity to develop. God's plan of perfection for the race can never be thwarted no matter how blindly we go astray. If we would shorten the period of our probation and trial, we must recognize the Truth of Being, and work with the law of constant unfoldment and developing improvement. There is a divine discontent that spurs us onward and upward, but far from being incompatible with poise and confidence and trust it is furthered by these; and it is wide as the poles asunder from fret and worry and anxiety.

Our problem is to adjust the outer man, the physical self, to harmonious relations with his inner spiritual self; for this is the only path to the overcoming of temptations, folly, and disease,— all the evils in short which purely physical or material living generates. The right use of the power of thought is the medium of adjustment, and we choose for ourselves what use shall be made of it. When an evil thought enters the mind promptly replace it with a good one. This is much better than to engage in a struggle to resist evil. It is the quickest method of shunting the mind to another track and of shutting the door between you and temptation, if the evil be of that nature. And at the same time it strengthens the mind to admit only the good, and trains desire to long for it and choose it. You thus cultivate receptivity to the highest, the best, and the purest; and are constantly refining and harmonizing the vibrations in every sphere of your being.

I wish to impress upon every reader the overwhelming importance of realizing individual responsibility for the perfection of the physical body,— the soul's medium of expression. It is in our power to steadily improve and purify these bodies of ours through the renewing materials we supply them. It is a significant sign of the times that Congress has at last passed a Pure Food bill. For years, highly protected interests have defeated all efforts to obtain legislation for this protection of the people, but a few stout hearts have kept up the fight till they roused such force of public opinion to support them that legislators no longer dared defy completely the will of the people. But pure foods and drinks are not enough. The world at large needs to recognize that pure air and pure thoughts as well as pure environment — the people and things forming our associations and moulding our tastes — are even more important than what we shall eat and drink.

To make these physical tenements receptive to the subtle vibrations of higher planes of activity — that is higher human development — we cannot be too careful concerning the materials in all these varied forms which they are constantly assimilating. Let not a day pass that you do not aspire for the highest and best things in the mental and the spiritual life,— for more "Light on the Path," and for steadfastness of purpose in pursuing it;

remembering always that *the Path is within!* in your choice of every thought and act.

The parts of the body through which the higher Principles operate lie in juxtaposition to the spine or are immediately connected therewith, and herein lies the supreme importance of the special exercises in Concentration by means of which we gain the power to rouse the *Kundalini,* and raise the latent, "coiled-up" energy through the *Sushumnâ;* the opening of which even a little way marks a distinct advance in spiritual and mental power, and in the overcoming of the physical.

Along the line of the *Sushumnâ* are ranged the seven *padmas,* or "*lotuses*" of the Yogi, stations, as it were, in the path of progress from the physical to the spiritual, which correspond with the principal nerve-plexuses from the basic, or sacral, to the pineal gland. In the head are seven "Master *Chakras*" which are said to govern and rule these nerve-plexuses in the body. Exactly in the proportion that the *Kundalini* is raised in the *Sushumnâ* the power of the current increases; for it stimulates every plexus as it passes through it, and also gathers to itself a tremendous increase from the essence or energy of the successive plexuses.

This force of supernormally pure and subtle vibrations reacts upon the whole nervous system, vastly increasing the power (through refining the vibrations) of every ganglion and strengthening and stimulating the zodiacal centers of the higher Principles. In this practice for Concentration, deep, slow rhythmic breathing should be so established that it will take care of itself. A mental image should be formed of the upward flow of the vital current. You must endeavor to both feel and see it rising in the *Sushumnâ* in obedience to your command, and gaining force as it ascends.

Leo, the zodiacal house of the sun, corresponds with and is the influence which develops life,— the vital force which we know as *Prâna*. But the form which that life-principle shall mould depends upon the character of our thoughts. The thought-principle, as you have learned, develops under the influence of Sagittarius. In the circle of the Zodiac, Sagittarius is on the same plane with Leo (life), but it is its opposite and complement, marking the immense evolution from mere animal life to the development of conscious mentality; and it stands, as explained in the last chapter, at the parting of the ways. If brought under a soul-governed Will, it leads the life, through the development of individuality to the upward arc of evolution, the divine quaternary,— to the release of the soul from its physical chains forged by sense-perceptions.

Individuality has its physical seat in the spine back of the heart, and is under the influence of Capricornus, always recognized as possessing a mysterious organizing power. Capricornus is on the boundary line of the manifested, or visible universe. On this gross plane of the physical man the constellation rules the knees. When you say of a man, "He is weak-kneed," you are unconsciously recognizing his lack of development in the Occult center of Capricornus, where, as individuality increases, courage keeps pace with it in the high council-chamber of the heart.

The correspondence of Leo with the body is through the solar plexus and the heart. The solar plexus (also called epigastric plexus) is to the nervous system what the heart is to the vascular system; therefore, it claims pre-eminence as the most vital center in the body. It is the largest of the great sympathetic plexuses, and is situated in the upper part of the abdomen, back of the stomach and in front of the aorta. Its dominating influence has won for it the titles of "abdominal brain" and "king brain." In this life-center, the three *Tattvas* which predominate in our terrestrial lives mingle most closely, and exercise the one upon the other that restraint which secures their harmonious co-operation in physical activities. *Prithivi* here unites with *Tejas*, and both come under the tempering, welding influence of *Âpas*, resolving them into a higher power. Remember the solvent and contracting properties of *Âpas*. These act with beneficent restraint upon the two others; therefore, concentration upon the solar plexus has an immediate effect in calming and purifying the nerves and restoring the equilibrium. It is the most important center upon which to concentrate for relief from any disturbance of the digestive function, whether gastric or intestinal.

Next above Capricornus in the circle of the Zodiac, is the zodiacal influence of the soul, Aquarius. The physical correspondence of this constellation is with that part of the spinal cord situated between the shoulders. Reference has already been made to the mystic relations between *Āpas* (water) and the soul, and this makes still clearer the bond between the two. Soul is that Principle in all things which relates the visible to the invisible; and in humanity it is the real, immortal Self,— the garment of the Spirit. It is that principle of universal love which makes the whole world kin. All self-sacrifice and self-forgetfulness in devotion to high principle is a manifestation of the soul. Only by such exercise does the soul come into conscious government of its own individual kingdom,— a conquest which must precede all realization of its oneness with infinite life and with power.

You must now have learned past forgetting that our bodies are the fields of marvellously subtle activities which, by reflection and transmutation from one plane to another lower one, are gradually precipitated into the visible form that constitutes the physical self. But never is there any separation. These activities are wheels within wheels; spheres within spheres. Also, you know that these *Tattvic* vibrations can be evil as well as beneficent; and that thought is the dynamic power which controls the vibrations, and can *make them whatever you choose!*

The relations of mind and body as you must certainly recognize by this time, are so intimate that the control of one is indispensable for the control of the other; for the mind really moulds the body from moment to moment through the instant effect of its every emotion upon the vibratory currents active therein, which are beneficent or evil according to the direction given them by habitual thoughts.

When you are told that the speed of the spirillæ within the atoms is " several hundred trillion " vibrations per second, the fact may help you to understand why intense emotion thrills the body so instantaneously and is capable of killing or curing according to its nature.

The ordinary every-day life which is absorbed with purely utilitarian occupations,— the life which is allowed to drift, and honestly believes it has no time to think purposefully,— wastes an incalculable force daily and hourly in ungoverned thinking and idle talking, and is fortunate when it does not suffer physical weakness and discord as a direct and speedy consequence. Many headaches, attacks of indigestion, and even colds (following mental depression) have no other origin than talk which, waxing into controversy, develops irritation, heated excitement and unhappiness.

You are now at a stage in this study of Self and its forces where you can readily understand that exercises in Concentration should always conclude with concentration upon the higher centers, and with an upward direction of currents, as these are psychical and spiritual, while downward-flowing currents are physical.

Never allow the body to become tense and strained during concentration; and avoid gazing fixedly at any object as a help in centering the mind. The practice (frequently commended) strains and injures the optic nerves, impairing their power of focal adjustment. As directed in an early chapter, it is much better to close the eyes when concentrating; and when the immediate purpose of the exercise is to restore physical harmony, confine consciousness — the inward gaze — as far as possible unwaveringly to the chosen center.

I think it must be clearly understood now that these exercises in Concentration are not to be considered from a purely utilitarian standpoint, the gain in physical well-being. No; the reward is far greater than that. It is a development, a remoulding on a higher plane, of the whole character, strengthening and giving firmness to every good quality, and disclosing talents and abilities before unsuspected. Harmony and serenity become the habitual mental state, and a source of unvarying courage and confidence in every perplexity and emergency. Thus we are moulding the Self to loftier purpose, to greater usefulness, to activities subliminal as well as conscious that affect for great good ourselves and all who come within our environment.

CHAPTER XX

THE CROWN OF CONCENTRATION

So far all the explanations concerning exercises and discipline for concentration have necessarily given prominence to the physical plane, because we must know our mediums of activity in order to use them correctly and beneficially; and because the physical is the lowest and grossest medium in the scale of human development, but also the vehicle of expression for all activities, and therefore the one which we must first learn to control.

No method of purifying and energizing the nerves is known to Western science that in any respect approaches the efficacy of the exercises for *Prânâyâma;* and from their effect upon the vibrations, they prepare the physical conditions most favorable for success in higher concentration.

In the *Sushumnâ* man bridges the abyss between the physical and spiritual over the psychic realm. It is only through the complete mastery of our thoughts and their conscious direction to the highest and best that we are able to open this gateway to the inner senses; for the process refines the vibrations of normal consciousness so that they are attuned to those of the supernormal state,— variously described as "subliminal," "The Unconscious Mind," and "The Subconscious." As it is a vastly higher condition, not lower, supernormal seems to identify it most clearly and aptly. Consciousness really embraces all space, which is to it non-existent; want of affinity in vibrations is the only bar. Therefore there are no limitations to the consciousness of the "knower." Ignorance or choice forge their own limitations of condition or state. Thus this normal self which we know best is commonly a person of many limitations because failing to utilize its latent powers. As long as we permit our desires to dwell upon lower physical pleasures this gateway remains closed, the thought-power needed to open it being wasted and dissipated in the world of externality. Passing downward and outward it brings deterioration of character, and effectually blocks the development of higher Principles.

I would entreat you to keep this basic fact ever before you as both a warning and a guide: The law of growth and development is based upon activity, and the form of the activity upon the use to which we devote it. No growth is possible without use; and just as every unused muscle or tightly bound organ in the body deteriorates through the stagnation thus induced, so also do unused faculties of the human mind deteriorate; while some powers remain ever latent from utter failure to exercise them.

Activity in a center quickens the sensitiveness of that center to receive impressions and to develop its latent powers. The spiritual nature within all is striving for unfoldment, and thus it is with every latent quality or power. It waits only the unlocking of its secret chamber through command of desire and searching intelligence. The weak-willed are governed by their desires excited by external objects; the strong-willed *govern their desires through internal choice*,— the ethical exercise of a discriminating will.

In the heart-silence to which concentration leads, sources of power undreamed-of are opened to us. The clear realization by the conscious self of conditions — fields of activity — usually veiled by subconsciousness, is developed through the increased activity of the soul when thus freed, and of a will-power which becomes in its every exercise a manifestation of soul-force. Not till we thus unite our wills with our real selves can we have any conception of the might of the invisible into whose realms we are gradually and gently led through this concentration of psychic power and consequent development of psychic senses. The keenness of these on the subtle planes where alone they act is another incontestable proof of the building power of the imaging faculty. Never idle, always moulding something, through its wise direction we can consciously enter the higher planes.

One of the earliest signs of progress in overcoming — in refining and purifying the vibrations — and in the unfoldment of the higher Principles, is the development of the sense of touch to a marvelously delicate rapport with the mind. It thus imparts to all abstract concepts whatsoever, of things as of persons, so intense reality that you discriminate textures and substances as if in actual contact with them; and can feel the presence of an absent friend — the really vital, throbbing life; the cordial handclasp or loving touch upon the hair — as vividly as if you stood face to face. The sense of smell also, always mysteriously linked with memory and subtly uniting us with the invisible, increases in sensitiveness to the stimulant of suggestion, promptly responding by presenting to consciousness the spiritual aroma of any favorite flower. The emotional effect of the sense of smell and the marvelous reactionary power of memory to stimulate it may be accounted for by its anatomical seat in close association with the pineal gland.

Not surprsing is it, therefore, that the first of the psychic senses to develop is the enjoyment of the spiritual aromas of Nature, — sweet flower-odors and aromatic pines and balsams which penetrate consciousness unpreparedly and in places where the physical vehicle of the odor is entirely absent. Its corresponding physical sense is stimulated, you will remember, by the last and densest *Tattva, Prithivi*, the earth vibration. It was the last sense to be evolved. Thus psychic evolution is exactly the reverse of physical evolution. It is the ascension of the spiral and reflects its opposite.

Corresponding with taste is the psychic power to absorb and enjoy the finer essences of *Prâna;* and to recall with the vividness of physical pleasure any delicious food flavors. These subtle essences are the nectar and ambrosia of the gods.

It is in the exercise of holding consciousness to the fixed contemplation of the force circulating in the *Sushumnâ* till it rises to the pineal gland and rouses it to activity, that the Yogi, in Swâmi Vivekânanda's words: " Becomes *en rapport* with the astral light and the universal mind and thus is able to see the whole Kosmos." All that is known of the invisible universe has been learned in this way. Physiological facts are these: When we succeed in rousing the *Kundalini*, and the vital-current rises in the *Sushumnâ*, we have released *Prâna* from its bondage to matter — that is, the nervous system, over which its currents normally flow — and in doing this have refined the vibrations to a higher plane to which it carries Consciousness with it. Thus we release the mind from its physical chains, the nerve-wires, and from the restrictions of the physical senses. The same principal is employed in wireless telegraphy!

The pineal gland is the "Divine Eye," and it is now recognized by scientists as "a vestigial structure representing an unpaired eye"; that is, the "third eye." Dr. Oliver Wendell Holmes described this mysterious organ as a small mineral deposit of grape-like masses of crystalline matter in the core of the brain, "in the part where Des Cartes placed the soul." Quantities of nerve fiber pass through the organ, and it is of interest to the student of the *Tattvas* to learn that of its two sorts of cells, those of sharp, irregular form contain granules of yellow or orange pigment. The macrocosmic correspondence of this gland is with Aries, and consciousness is there enthroned.

The structure of the pituitary body is almost identical with that of the pineal gland, yet no slightest connection can be traced between the two centers by anatomists. Mme. Blavatsky is my authority, however, for stating that the connection between them is physiological as well as spiritual. Her assertions concerning their importance were corroborated in 1903 by the discoveries of Dr. Sajous, of Philadelphia, who announced the "startling theory that one of the least studied glands [the pituitary body] is the most important of the millions in the human body." After fourteen years of research devoted especially to the study of the office or function of the least understood glands in the body, Dr. Sajous believed he could demonstrate that the anterior lobe of the pituitary body [of course, the difference between the lobes is that one is positive and the other negative] is vitally concerned in the preservation of health, *because the glands are agents for the absorption of oxygen and its transmission in another form to the lungs.* When you study the sheaths of the body, this discovery will strike you with greater significance.

Concerning the connection between the pituitary body and the pineal gland, Mme. Blavatsky states that an Adept can see a golden aura pulsating in both centers when the subject is in a *normal* condition. It is as regular as the heart beat. Under abnormal conditions of concentration or exaltation, the arc of pulsation from the pituitary body mounts upward more and more until, just as when an electric current strikes some solid object, the vibrations strike the pineal gland, and awakening that dormant center set all glowing with pure *Âkâshic* energy.

" This is the psycho-physiological illustration of two organs on the physical plane, which are respectively, the concrete symbols of the metaphysical concepts called *Manas* [mind] and *Buddhi* [Soul]. To become conscious on this plane, *Buddhi* needs the differentiated fire of *Manas;* but *once the sixth sense has awakened the seventh* the light which radiates from this seventh sense illuminates the fields of infinitude. For a brief space of time, man becomes omniscient, the Past and the Future, Space and Time, disappear and become for him the Present."

Thus experience, as tangible and definite as any scientific experiments, has established the fact that the pineal gland is the chief organ of spirituality, and the seat of genius. It is the "concrete symbol" because latent within this crystalline center are the potencies of *Buddhi.* To the faithful earnest student, it becomes the magical Sesame which under the stimulus of his purified will opens to him the secrets of the macrocosm. This supreme achievement, however, is not the reward of all, nor can it be gained by any without unfaltering purpose.

Any selfish aim defeats the realization of higher states of consciousness. But all faithful and regular practice brings its immediate return in serenity, mental power, and physical harmony; with a steady gain in these day by day, and increasing strength, insight, and confidence. Always, the purer the thoughts, the finer, the more rapid the vibrations of the mind-stuff whose reflection is mirrored upon the physical plane.

Know, too, that spiritual consciousness cannot

be taken by assault. It can be won only by persevering, patient devotion to the lofty purpose of union with the highest. It requires effort and continuous effort, and especially the self-discipline of restraining all irritation or depression. Boundless faith, cheerfulness and happiness create those harmonious vibrations that prepare the lower sheaths to reflect the higher, and release subtle forces to pass freely from one medium to another. No other investment of time or labor returns so soul-satisfying, enduring rewards.

To see the vision, and without striving and hoping for it none can succeed, one must "think inwardly; desire intensely; and imagine centrally;" resolved that nothing shall bar one's penetrating to the innermost radiant center of being — the Living Temple — and ascending to the highest, most subtle plane. By concentration, the diffused, latent soul-power is made manifest and definite,— comprehensible. Meditation is the crown of concentration. It is only in meditation that we reach the heart of anything. We cannot meditate till through concentration we have brought the medium, the mind, to the steadfast state of submission to our will and purpose. Thus concentration is the moulding of the organ; meditation is its exercise to great ends.

The first successful stage is to be able to hold the mind to a single point; and next to sweep the surface clean of any object; literally to fix the attention upon nothing. This is the "waveless lake" of Swâmi Vivekânanda,— a clean tablet upon which, having brought the mind-stuff into a state of perfect quiescence, we can pursue a single train of thought; each link in the chain, by the law of causation which is also a law of rhythm, rising into consciousness and taking its place with the precision of well-trained soldiers.

Do not confound concentration with a state of passivity. In order to reach the plane of pure meditation which opens the channels for an influx of divine power,— where, as Annie Besant says: "Peace and strength and force flow into the soul,"— it is necessary to quell all the distractions of irrelevant ideas with which the senses and untrained minds commonly make havoc of lives. These most certainly must be reduced to a state of passivity, hence the confusion; but if consciousness be permitted to dwell upon this plane, the result is not *concentration but stupor!* This is the mistake, the stumbling-block in many paths.

Consciousness must ascend; through aspiration it must be alert yet not anxious. It must concentrate all effort to a single point. Thus it is a state of highest activity. The master on duty cannot sleep! The only danger incurred in the exercise is from excessive zeal. The subtle vibrations called into activity work through the germs of the powers you seek to develop; and, like all life in its incipiency, these germs — atomic spirillæ — are extremely delicate. Practice should always stop short of brain-fatigue.

The earnest student needs no admonition; but the curious investigator who experiments with this system of unfoldment and evolution is cautioned that the mental attitude with which the study is pursued affects most profoundly the results. The poison of doubt, or any lack of confidence acts effectively to inhibit the realization of the benefits sought. Trust and hopefulness open the channels for their fulfillment. Be not too keen for results. That attitude easily passes into anxiety and disappointment. It is to the cheerfully expectant that all great boons come. Let your greatest interest be in the method; in the difficulties you encounter, and the ingenuity, the expedients, you evolve in overcoming them. Remember that you are investigating your own kingdom of consciousness; a mysterious realm that will open out gradually, disclosing resources, possibilities, and talents wholly unsuspected.

Do not dwell upon things external. It is *within* you must endeavor to center all your consciousness. Give no recognition to insistent sense-perceptions; *ignore everything external.* Not by denial of what obtrudes persistently, for that implies recognition, but by steadfast affirmation of what you seek will you reach the goal of endeavor — complete abstraction from the material, visible plane. The forces that ingather during such concentration are commonly wasted in prodigal outward radiation; for there is more spendthrift thinking than there is spendthrift waste of money. Not till the psychic force which is commonly squandered so thoughtlessly and lavishly is gathered in and concentrated in various centers does the normal consciousness realize the extent to which the power can be controlled, or the energy which can be thus generated.

Above all, during the exercise of concentration, the mind should not be permitted to dwell for an instant upon the anxieties, vicissitudes, or annoyances of the day. It should be lifted to the consciousness of eternal peace,—the law of the perfectly adjusted life. The first stage of the subjective, interior self which we reach in the Silence, is that most closely connected with normal consciousness where the effects of habitual thoughts and acts are garnered and reproach or comfort us according to their nature; and in the degree that we are able to make this self-examination with absolute candor and freedom from bias or prejudice, is it helpful to us. Do not tarry here; waste no time in regret; give only such recognition as arms you against repetition of that which harms. Harmonious thoughts alone can mould a harmonious body, and desire for things spiritual can alone give the real self opportunity to grow and to evolve its inherent power.

It is a deeply significant truth that the regular observance of periods for Concentration produces physical and mental conditions that favor such development beyond any other known discipline or training. Only during introspection, after complete withdrawal from the world of the senses, has the soul-life an opportunity to strengthen itself through association with things spiritual and subjective, instead of material and objective. Every such exercise of the soul-life refines and purifies the vibrations and reflects its increasing strength and purity upon the physical tabernacle.

For, mystery of mysteries! it is into the realm of creation that meditation carries us, where we feel the dawning of a creative spirit in ourselves; and realize beyond question or faintest doubt that we, too, can share in that higher life,— that we are a part of it and can manifest our individual part here.

CHAPTER XXI

THE SEQUENCE OF NUMBERS

ONE of the most significant and deepest truths of life, of Nature, of the Universe, is, that there is correspondence — fundamental correspondence — everywhere. The stumbling-block of science has been its separation of man, the observer, from the objects of his study and research; for he, the crowning work of creation, is an epitome of it, bearing to its component parts the same relations that the atoms of his body bear to one another.

It is impossible for us to separate ourselves from the life about us, for we are a part of it, and bear the closest relationship to its manifold forms and manifestations. The soul, the connecting link between the body and its Creator, is the medium through which all consciousness of that Divinity and our close connection with the unchanging source of life is manifested. Now, the question arises: How is it manifested?

You have been told that everything, all activity, every visible thing, is the result of *Tattvic* vibrations; and that our physical bodies are gross —

that is, *visible* — effects of their ceaseless permutations and comminglings. The distinction "gross" is used in this connection always with the sense of being the antipodes, or direct opposite of the most sublimated or subtle,— a visible effect, through a succession of ever coarsening vibrations forming denser matter, of invisible forces; forces of so tremendous energy that the average mind is as yet incapable, wanting any standard of comparison, of realizing their power and effect. What you have already learned concerning the bonds of sympathy established by the *Tattvas* has prepared you for the consideration now of all the links in the chain of causation, the analysis of which will enable you to answer in fullest detail and incontrovertibly the question: What is this relationship and correspondence? in answering which the first question is answered also.

All this is made clear through study of the Self, — a septenary compound of Principles which link the microcosm to the macrocosm by the same septenary chain through and by which all phenomena issue from the noumenon. The human body consists of seven vehicles of expression,— sheaths, bodies, or Principles, as they are variously designated. The lowest of these in degree of density is the physical body, an aggregation of cells compounded by the grossest vibrations of the *Tattvas;* but cells could not exist without molecules, nor molecules without atoms; and just as every process from the exterior to the interior of the cell is a gradation of refining motion, to forms and vibrations too subtle for the comprehension of man, so also is the structure of the human body.

The sequence of numbers forges the links in this life-chain,— numbers ever repeating, ever reiterating, ever reproducing and recombining — constrained by the Rhythmic Law — the primary Logoi emanating from the First Cause. As from this First Cause, which is Unity (the Creator, Brahman), everything in the manifested world proceeds, the basic Truth is that the Law of Unity is the keystone of the arch supporting, defining, and limiting all other laws and their activities. But since manifestation implies change, how does this Law of Unity act? Every act proceeds from an impelling influence,— the *power of thought, which is Spirit in action*. God thought, and instantly the vibrations of that thought — for us the first manifestation of Force — began working in its affinity, or opposite, the Mother Principle of the Universe, *Mûla-prakriti;* or *Pradhâna;* homogeneous, undiscrete substance for which there are many names. It suffices for clearest understanding, however, to recognize it as the *negative* phase of Spirit, and the root of matter, which is always negative to Spirit.

Thus even Unity *in action* must have two phases

— activity and existence being unthinkable, otherwise — and these two aspects of the First Cause are necessarily of different character, opposite poles the one to the other, hence give rise to diversity in Unity; whence arises the law of affinity, or sympathy, in opposites. Therefore, " pairs of opposites " are to be held in mind as the basis of all activities, all change, all progress, and the beginning of numbers,— the duad, without which the Holy Trinity were impossible. Affinity is the Love Principle which builds all worlds, while its opposite, hate, destroys. The opposite of unity is diversity, and the product of their interaction is a unit which differs from them,— the Trinity, the three in one, or three aspects of the Primary Cause. The very beginning of Kosmic manifestation was an unfolding of this three-fold power, the Trinity, which was latent in Unity. To put this in simple terms of every day life which should speak to every human heart in a voice that will forever echo the truth: Father, mother, and child are forever reiterating, reproducing the Primary activity of the Holy Trinity.

These aspects are defined in Principles as Will, Wisdom, and Activity,— the Will *to do*, the Wisdom *to conceive*, the Power *to act*. The ideas of all created things are inherent in this first utterance of Supreme Unity, which we recognize as the First Logos,— the expression or Voice of God, who spoke the Universe into existence; for the resulting vibrations are the Holy Spirit or creative medium. This First Logos was seven-fold, and differentiated into the seven Logoi, or creative potencies, (the Seven Spirits, or gods, below the Trinity), corresponding to the vowels of speech, and acting through the septenary of vowel-sounds. Thus sound and color and form correspond throughout Nature.

In the "*Book of Dzyan*" (see *Secret Doctrine*, Vol. I.), it is said: "This was the army of the Voice — The Divine Septenary. . . . These are called spheres, triangles, cubes, lines, and modellers." You will recognize these forms as identical with the *Tattvas*, and it shows you that from the beginning of manifestation God geometrized. The Harmony of the Spheres, Pythagoras' "Voice of Nature," is composed of these voices of the Logoi, which correspond with the seven tones of the musical scale. They are the seven heavens, or angels, who "sounded each one vowel, which, all combined together, formed a complete doxology;" the *Sound* whereof, being carried down to earth, "became the creator and parent of all things that be on earth." The forces thus set in motion are the Seven Hierarchs of conscious divine powers, active manifestations of one Supreme Energy. In Hindu mythology, this stage of evolution is known as "the creation of the gods," the sons of Fohat, or Force. These personified forces are the positive aspects of the *Tattvas*, the negative phases being the *Shaktis* of the Hindu *Sacred Books*.

Now, the Logoi must be recognized also as " the Seven Great Rays " from the Holy Spirit, or Primal Light. It is these seven Forces, symbolized as the " Elohim or Seven Spirits of God "— the lower Sephiroth of the Kabala — which define the limits to the links in the chain of causation, establishing seven planes of manifestation, corresponding each with its primal Ray and its vowel sound, and differentiated the one from the others by the character of its vibrations; that is, their form and rate, or number per unit of time — their velocity.

The Western mind has little idea of the latent power in sound and consequently in words, numbers, and musical tones. But number underlies all form and guides sound. All life is manifested in numerical proportions and rhythmical motion. Motion, ceaseless motion is a condition of all existence, and form determines its effect; but sound with its rhythm and accent, of which number is the expression, *moulds the form*. Thus, the Voice of God — sound — shaped the vibrations of the First Logos which contained in itself the germs of the succeeding seven Logoi.

It is, perhaps, fortunate that we are forced to

employ the Sanskrit nomenclature for the *Tattvas;* because Sanskrit being a pure, primitive tongue, is rich in onomatopoetic words like our cool, fiery, rustling, brilliant, scurry. There is great probability that the names of the *Tattvas* bear a metrical relation to their signification, quality, and action on the gross plane of matter. Hence it is very important that they be correctly pronounced. To facilitate this, the accepted phonetic spelling (that adopted by the Sanskrit scholars who appreciate the need) has been strictly followed; and to give further aid a glossary of all the Sanskrit words it has been necessary to use is appended to this book.

The marvellous building and formative power in sound has always been recognized in Hindu religion and philosophy, and it has led the East Indian people to have an unshakable faith in the potency of their most sacred Word. They believe the manifestating Word of God is *Om* (*Aum*), and, being "double in its pronunciation and triple in its essence," that it expresses every power of generation, preservation, and destruction; that is, correspondence with their Trimurti (Trinity) — Brahma, the creator; Vishnu, the preserver; and Shiva, the destroyer; "all one in different aspects."

Although there are hundreds of words in different languages signifying God, there must be some root thought, generalization, or common ground from which all the symbols spring; and that root thought, "the primitive idea," reasons the Hindu, "should be the common symbol." He, therefore, seeks his fundamental in a root sound, asking himself first, how sounds are uttered by the human voice, and then, "What must have been the first sound?"

What organs are called into action? The larynx, and the palate as a sounding board. Now, is there any word which contains in itself the basis of all sounds? Yes, *Aum* (*Om* — pronounced like o in on, *not* like o in home, prolonging the consonant and holding the voice to one key) is such a word, and the *only one*. Analyzing its "triple essence," the first letter, *A,* is the root sound, or key. In all tongues, it is the natural exclamation of emotion, whether of pain or joy (ah!), and the first word the infant utters; and it is pronounced without touching any part of the tongue or palate. *U* rolls from the very root of the tongue to the end of the mouth's soundingboard; and *M* brings teeth and lips together and closes mouth and sound. The three letters also symbolize the three worlds, physical, astral (or luminous), and heavenly; the latter embracing the other two (see Glossary).

Thus, *Om* is a fundamental word covering the whole phenomena of vocal utterance. As such, Swâmi Vivekânanda pronounces it "the natural symbol, the matrix of all the various sounds," believing that "It denotes the whole range and possibility of all the words that can be made." All the religious ideas of India have been and are centered around this sacred Word; so hallowed in many cults that its public utterance has been condemned when not forbidden. And this ban you will now understand arises from no mere superstition but is based upon Occult knowledge of the tremendous power invested in certain rhythmic sounds. I would caution you never to utter the word or discuss its profound significance in hostile or flippant company; "because," says Annie Besant, "the sound that, working in the harmonious builds, working in the inharmonious destroys; and every thing that is evil is tumultuous, while everything which is pure is harmonious" (*Building of the Kosmos*, p. 23).

A Sanskrit *Mantra* embodies in its words an essential virtue attributed to the rhythmic force of sound; and Mrs. Besant, addressing the Theosophical Society, in India, explained that she used the "teaching" of the Upanishad *(Mundako)* but not the "Sanskrit tongue in the definite order of its syllables which gives them the force of *Mantrams*." She would not assume the responsibility "of repeating the *Mantram*-form" of Vedic *Shlokas* in a mixed assembly where conflicting magnetisms were gathered.

I have dwelt thus upon the importance of the

spoken word as a caution to those thoughtless persons who frequently hold up to ridicule sacred words and subjects concerning the significance of which they are profoundly ignorant; and doing which they make for themselves very unhappy Karma,— that unerring law which adjusts effect to cause on every plane,— which *their companions* and all those whom they influence share to a lesser degree. It is impossible to speak with too great emphasis here, for idle talk does more harm than the average mind can conceive; and hasty speech, the word that hurts, has ever to be atoned for. Forces that are uncontrolled, control *you;* and out of this mystery emanates all the suffering and unhappiness in the world. Choose ye harmonious forces.

Pythagorean philosophy taught that the substances of all things were represented by abstract numbers, which in a certain sense were the elements of the Universe and explained it. Every number, therefore, had its specific value and influence; and the Pythagoreans considered seven, or the *heptagon,* a religious and perfect number. It is called *Telesphorus* " because by it all in the Universe and mankind is led to its end "; and also, " because within the decade it has neither factors nor product." Plutarch says that Pythagoras maintained " the earth was the product of the cube; fire, of the pyramid (triangle?) ; air, of the octahedron; and the sphere of the Universe, of the dodecahedron." When you recognize the agreement between this theory and the *Tattvic* Law (in the form of elemental vibrations) you will, perhaps, think with me that the moderns would better cease to scoff at the " fantastic metaphysics " of Pythagoras, and with humble spirit and open minds study his tenets.

The number system of Pythagoras was based on the theory of opposites (by which alone Creation and the activities of the Kosmos can be explained). Numbers were divided into odd and even, and from their combination other numbers (and therefore all things) resulted. He believed number was the basis of order and harmony in the Kosmos, identified it with form; and endowed different numbers with their special virtues and powers.

The Pythagorean categories, or fundamental opposites are:

1. Limited and unlimited.
2. Odd and even.
3. One and many.
4. Right and left.
5. Masculine and feminine.
6. Rest and motion.
7. Straight and crooked.
8. Light and darkness.
9. Good and evil.
10. Square and oblong.

The first four numbers corresponded respectively with a point, a line, a surface, and a cube. The point (1) signified unity and harmony, or order, having position, and being analogous to the *monad* (Spirit, or Ego), was positive and bi-sexual, the number of origin and of reason; the line (2) was analogous to the *duad,* an even number, unlimited, because it could be perpetually halved, negative and feminine; and represented matter — therefore the possibility of evil — and brute force; a surface (3) was analogous to the *triad,* or triangle, positive and masculine; and a cube (4) to the *tetrad,* or Tetraktys; considered the symbol of the Kosmos, because containing within itself the point, the line, the superficies, and the solid — all essentials of form. Its mystical representation is the point within the triangle. Four was also significant as the first square number, and as being the potential decade (1+2+3+4=10), or perfect number. Pythagoras compared four to "a world that is self-moving; it contains in itself, and is, the quarternary." It was the number of justice, as was three of mediation.

Great honor was shown to three by all ancient peoples, as, corresponding with the triangle, it was the first absolutely perfect figure; endowed with sacred significance as symbolizing the Eternal, the first Perfection, and the three kingdoms. Although the science of good and evil began with two,

The Sequence of Numbers

which expresses all the contrasts in Nature — day and night, health and sickness, heat and cold, light and darkness, etc.— it yet was recognized as intimately connected with harmonic sound, "because by doubling the number of string vibrations in a given unit of time another tone is produced which *sounds* like the first, but differs in pitch — the octave higher."

Five was called "the nourisher,"— the generating and fostering sound; for it was believed that a fifth was the first of all intervals which could be sounded; and also it contained the first feminine or even number (2), and the first masculine or odd (3). Pythagoras discovered that the fifth and the octave of a tone could be produced on the same string by stopping at two-thirds and one-half of its length respectively. This gave the law that harmony depends upon numerical proportion, and the discovery is believed to have led to his whole philosophy of number.

The *Ogdoad* or eight symbolizes the eternal and spiral motion of all things from the atom to cycles, and is symbolized in its turn by the caduceus. It manifests the regular in-and-out-breathing of the Kosmos under the direction of the "eight great gods"— that is, the seven Builders or Kosmic Dhyan Chohans (identified with the "Seven Spirits," the "Voices," and the "Seven Angels of the Stars"), and the Holy Spirit, whence they emanated. Nine is the triple ternary, a number reproducing itself incessantly under all shapes and figures in multiplication. It is the sign of every circumference. It leads to a new dispensation and to revelation and symbolizes the point of union with the Higher Self. Under certain conditions, by the law of opposites, it may be very unlucky.

Ten, or the Decade, brings the digits back to unity and completes the Pythagorean table. Hence the figure 1. enclosed in a cipher — unity within zero — was a symbol of Deity, of the visible Universe and of infinite vastness, and of man, the only creature who stood erect; as also of the primal activity of the positive and negative forces. In the *Books of Hermes*, which Mme. Blavatsky quotes *(Secret Doctrine*, Vol. III.), *ten* is "the Mother of the Soul, Life and Light being therein united," for *one*, man, is born of the Spirit, and *ten*, of matter, and from their unity — again the Trinity — comes forth the Soul.

There is a famous Chinese arithmetical diagram called the *Loh-Shu*, or the scroll of the river *Loh;* the invention of which is attributed to Fuh-Hi who lived 2858-2738 B. C. It is a mathematical square from 1-9, so written that all the odd numbers are expressed in *yang* symbols,— white dots, emblems of heaven; while the even numbers are expressed in *yin* symbols,— black dots, the emblems of earth. Confucius, who was a contemporary of Pythagoras, used these same *yang* and *yin* symbols, with the already age-honored signification above given; and he taught that the transmutations and comminglings of these odd and even numbers — corresponding, of course, with forces — kept "the spirit-like agencies" of the Kosmic world in movement.

Thus the theory of opposites and of the fundamental relations of odd and even numbers was not confined to a brotherhood of "fantastic metaphysicians" in Greece, and is perhaps worthy of the serious consideration of modern scientists. The twentieth century has not improved upon the Confucian Code of Ethics, and ancient wisdom is a vast storehouse of treasures for us.

The seven-fold permutations of the *Tattvas* was explained early in these lessons (Chapter VI), but you are now to understand that everything in Nature responds to this number seven,— a compound of three and four, and the factor element in every ancient religion, *because it is the factor element in Nature*. The most tremendous and baffling force in Nature is the mysterious synthesizing power of the triad, the "three in one." It is the Unity which in all the apparent confusion maintains harmony and order. This synthetic power is shared in only lesser degree by five and seven, and these three are most significant numbers for humanity.

246 The Law of the Rhythmic Breath

Seven is "the master of the moon" for she is constrained to change her phase every seven days. Thus she herself is *without the seven*, being acted upon by them.

Mme. Blavatsky says: "The seven planets are not limited to this number because the ancients knew no others, but simply because they were the primordial or primitive *houses* of the seven *Logoi*. There may be nine and ninety-nine other planets discovered — this does not alter the fact of these seven alone being sacred." What you know of planetary influences will enable you to recognize the "houses" as centers respectively of the separate creative forces, or Logoi.

Though invisible and inaudible to us in detail, the creative forces, in the form of rates of vibration which compound and dissociate the atoms and molecules, become in the synthesis of the whole audible to us on the material plane. The Chinese call it the "Great Tone," or Kung. It is the actual tonic of Nature, recognized by musicians as middle *Fa* on the piano.

Among the moderns, the great French genius, Balzac (recently classed with Napoleon and other history-makers of the nineteenth century among the *demi-fous*, or half-insane) was gifted with a Pythagorean insight into the mysteries of the Kosmos. He wrote: "There is a Number beyond which the impure cannot pass; the Number which is the limit of creation.

"The Unit was [is?] the starting-point of every product. . . . The Universe is the Unit in variety. Motion is the means; Number is the result. The end is the return of all things to the Unit, which is God."

CHAPTER XXII

THE SEVEN-FOLD CONSTITUTION OF HUMANITY

WE have seen that proceeding from Unity through its first uttered thought,— the Voice of God striking upon the waters of Life,— Kosmic vibrations varied by sound, motion, and number, and restrained by unison and harmony, are the base and order of the Universe.

Never lose sight of the basic law that Unity in action is dual,— that in this fact lies the axial point of creation, as also the endurance of the Universe; that right here, the ultimate of manifestation that man's intelligence can reach or comprehend, is the Fohat feeding the Great Dynamo which maintains the absolute rhythm of the Great Breath of all Life. On every hand we have proof of these two opposed but complementary forces in Nature.

The attraction and repulsion of these two phases of one substance — that is, the reciprocal activities of the positive and the negative, or the active and the passive — are the source of perpetual motion. While each phase is in its purest state, sympathy draws them together; when they are completely blended, *antipathy* results and they fly apart.

Thus satiety follows rapture and prepares the way for further rapture; the two phases ever building and disintegrating, mingling and separating.

This duality exists in every differentiality from the First Cause, and therefore in every atom. This is the first bond of union and sympathy, the *phase* of motion; it is this that maintains the conservation of energy; and the next is the form, like seeking like, fire feeding fire, water blending with water, oil with oil; and from every duad is derived a third, which is the synthesis of the triad.

As the seven sounds, the tones, or voices of the Logoi — emanations from the Holy Spirit of the Primal Trinity — define through their differentiations, the limits of causation and, therefore, the links in the chain; through their activities, they established corresponding planes of existence, or manifestation, which are called the sheaths of Brahman. It is Brahman,— the Creator who is undefinable,—" The one Breath of the whole Universe," who set these limits to creation; without whom there could be no life; and not till the souls of men realize this can they attain immortality.

Now, wherever God is — and He is everywhere — the possibility, the germ of development, of evolution, is present; and it is in this sense that it can be truly said, from the *Truti* to man, every atom is an epitome of the Universe, having its correspondence with the sheaths or planes. Consciousness is inherent in substance, therefore embodied in the atom which is the soul of the molecule, so that "every molecule in the Universe is able to feel and to obey after its kind,— the inorganic as well as the organic" *(Perfect Way,* p. 122).

Sir William Crooke's "protyle," the withinness of his dual atom, is a *Prithivic Vâyu* sheath of this synthesizing spiritual ray— the soul of every atom, of every created thing. It is for this reason that to sensitive souls, the souls awakened to the presence of the Spirit, the immanence of the God-presence becomes in all the secret haunts of nature an abiding fact ever present to their consciousness. Therefore, these enlightened ones see more, hear more, feel more, and receive more from intimate association with nature than those average folk whose chief characteristics are their gregariousness, their obtuseness to blatant noise, and their love of excitement — often indeed, their acute horror of being alone. They are afraid of the mystery of life which in silence knocks on the door of consciousness,— afraid because it has been clothed in terror when it should be radiant with beauty.

Western science is to-day ably corroborating all that the ancient religions and wisdom have affirmed concerning this septenary chain of creation, of involution and evolution. The telescope has revealed that the great globe of Jupiter is divided into a series of concentric shells showing variations of motion and character. The eye is able to look through these varying planes, or spheres within spheres; and an ideal picture of the spectacle, drawn by Garrett Serviss, curiously enough shows exactly six concentric rings surrounding the luminous central sphere. Now this central sphere is the "home" of the ruling Logoi,— the soul of the planet, which rules its function and emanations and sounds its key. Our own earth has its enveloping sheaths in like manner, and its radiant center, the Higher Ego (this is "The Glory clothing the Hidden Spirit"), which is positive to *all its sheaths* but negative to its Creator, Life Eternal! Our sun holds in synthesis all the planetary rays sending to every one its own.

The astronomical symbol of the earth is a disc with a cross stretched from center to circumference. Has the deep significance of this ever occurred to you? It symbolizes the earth-life of humanity; the soul crucified upon and within the four elements of the physical plane; earth, water, fire, and air,— the stimulators of the senses and, through them, of desire. The ancient Hindu symbol called the Svastika (really a world symbol, as it has been found everywhere) is a modification of the earth sign; and, explained exoterically, signifies manifested life coming out of the unmanifested; that is, the arms of the Greek cross bent at right angles symbolize the human soul on the wheel of life, held to its orbit by the circle (understood) of the Spirit,— the one and only source of all life. There is, however, a profounder symbology: The bent arms mark the soul's recognition of its oneness with spirit, and its determination to evolve out of the physical sheaths into synchronous vibration with the spiritual plane; hence into the state of spiritual consciousness. That is, to transform its cross into a crown! In all the oldest records, the cross was always within the circle, which symbolizes Divine Unity, time unending, and the omnipresence of the unrecognizable.

You are familiar already with the fact that there are seven descriptions of life-currents corresponding with the planets, and it will not be difficult for you to understand that these seven fundamental forces in Nature are also seven planes of being, which, as Mme. Blavatsky explains very clearly, " are seven states of consciousness in which man can live, think, remember, and have his being."

These different Principles, sheaths, or bodies have received many names in the different religions and philosophies of both the ancient world and the modern; and have been variously classified as to order. Any attempt to enumerate all these and to reconcile them would make a book in itself. The significant fact is that these different states have been recognized in all religions and every philoso-

The Seven-fold Constitution of Humanity

phy worthy of the name. The Christian Triad of body, soul, and spirit includes the whole septenary chain; but it has given currency to the common belief that man is only a triadic creature; so we speak of physical, mental, and spiritual selves.

The analysis here given does not change the familiar classification, but goes further — closer to the heart and truth of things, distinguishing other divisions; and showing how every Principle or sheath influences and interpenetrates the others. The septenary constitution of humanity is symbolized by a triangle surmounting a cube or square. In the cube, we have the ultimate of manifestation, containing as it does the possibilities of all variety, of every form, of all expression; all the elements in one, being the actual form of *Prithivi*, the earth vibration.

The cube represents the four different sheaths which make up the " natural body " of earth life. The two outer are the *Sthula-Sharira*, or gross body; and the *Sûkshma-Sharira*, or subtle body — the Etheric-double, which is the prototype and shadow of the *Sthula*, being the form round which the physical body is built; and in some of its appearances it is called the astral body. The *Sûkshma-Sharira* is the vehicle of *Prâna*, which is transmuted through the astral spleen, and thus the life-current unites the two bodies. The *nœuds-vital* in the throat and " the pit of the stomach," so-called (the great vagus nerve and the solar plexus), are the points of closest connection between these *Shariras,* which explains the sensitiveness of these physical centers. The restoration of those who have been shocked by electricity or smothered by drowning is effected through such stimulation of these centers as restores connection between these bodies and thus recalls the Ego to consciousness. This is the secret of the wonder-working *Kat-zu* (resuscitation from apparent death) of the Japanese. The remaining sheaths of the quarternary are the desire-body, or *Kâmarupa,* the principle which uncontrolled gives physical man the most trouble; and the animal soul, or mind, Lower *Manas.* Mme. Blavatsky describes the latter as "The reflection or shadow of the *Buddhi-Manas* [Higher *Manas*], but often conquered by *Kâmic* elements." She states farther: "There are enormous mysteries connected with Lower *Manas.* With regard to some intellectual giants, they are in somewhat the same condition as smaller men, for their Higher Ego is paralyzed; that is to say, their spiritual nature is atrophied" *(Secret Doctrine,* Vol. III, p. 592).

These sheaths of the quarternary, correspond as enumerated with the *Tattvas* from *Prithivi* to *Vâyu.*

The upper triad ascends through Higher *Manas,* Higher Ego, Causal Body, or *Kârana-Sharira*—

The Seven-fold Constitution of Humanity

various names for one sheath or principle; to Buddhi, the soul, or spiritual sheath; and terminates with the Auric Egg, or Âtma,— the Divine Spirit. The seventh holds all the other sheaths in synthesis; but the lower member of the triad, as in all trinities, holds the two highest Principles in synthesis and also, as the fifth from the lowest *Sharira*, holds the lower quartenary in synthesis, and unites them to the higher. You have doubtless recognized this as the all-pervading *Âkâsha*.

The two higher Principles, the duad of the upper triad (6–7), pervade everything in nature from the mineral upwards, but only in man is the fifth Principle found in an active state. It is the Causal Body, the beginning of individuality and consciousness, and marks the passage of the life from the beast to the human.

The four lower Principles are those in which, during earth life, the Spirit is involved; and the three higher, those through which by ascent the soul accomplishes its evolution — earns its immortality. Do not think of these sheaths or planes as one above another, either in the Universe or in man. All seven may be said to permeate all space. Their difference is a variation in form of manifestation of one and the same substance — Eternal Spirit; and this change in form is a change of velocity as well as change in combination of the primary simple *Tattvas*. The change is best and most simply described as increasing density and decrease of velocity from the highest to the lowest, which must be understood also as from inner to outer; or counting upwards from the lower and outer — that is, the physical body — the sheaths grow more subtle and the vibrations increase tremendously in velocity as they proceed from lowest to highest, from without to the radiant center of life. All these bodies change, deteriorate or improve, according to the materials we draw into them through our thoughts and emotions.

The rays of the Spirit radiate in every direction from the center to circumference, but the atoms of the separate sheaths are conditioned to the plane of their manifestation by the rates of their vibrations. These definite planes, or spheres, reflect one another as in a mirror; reflection proceeding downward and outward, every sheath being receptive to the next higher, and attracted to the next lower; but the Spirit radiates outward throughout the sheaths. Thus the Spirit is never in bondage to nature, even when working in and manipulating it; and the soul, the vehicle of the Spirit, has but to recognize its power in order to utilize it and manifest its freedom. *The light is always within;* but whether we reveal or obscure it depends upon the density of our outer spheres,— upon the character we are building for ourselves through our activities, tastes, and aims.

Thus man must master these forces or be mastered by them; and his whole task in life is the transmutation of lower forces into higher, whereby he may develop the spiritual forces within and come into conscious recognition of his soul,— his Higher Ego.

What chiefly concerns us, then, is to gain consciousness on the spiritual plane. It is only a question of seeking the highest, and compelling obedience from the horde of trivialities on the lower plane which commonly occupy our entire field of consciousness, holding us there with their insistent demands.

CHAPTER XXIII

COLOR IN THE VISIBLE AND INVISIBLE WORLD

Part I.

ALL that exists, the whole visible Universe, is a manifestation of Force, of vibratory energy differentiated not by velocity alone but by form; and every form has its color, as also its tone, or sound.

Thus certain colors are inseparably associated with certain forms of vibration, and, consequently, with conditions of substance. The *color is in the substance,* whether there be light by which to see it or all is darkness. For example: The potency of a drug or herb may be recognized by its color, and it will have exactly the same effect if administered in the dark as if taken in broadest daylight. Moreover, the form in which it is prepared may entirely conceal its normal color, for the great solvent *Âpas* (water) has the power to hold the color latently, but therein lies its power. In therapeutic color-treatment — chromopathy — the patient continues through the darkness of the night to receive the restorative harmonizing vibrations of the color by which he is surrounded; and the effect of that color is from its explicit action upon the human sheaths.

In chemical research, the hints which color gives are but half-understood, and throughout the scientific world its power and mystery are greatly depreciated. In the chemical changes of atoms, all variations of colors indicate fundamental differences in either their constitution or their phase,—whether positive or negative. Dr. Babbitt's investigations led him to conclude that the positive, or active, color was always within the atom, and the negative, or passive, without. But to my understanding this is only a half-truth, describing one atomic phase; and it is not corroborated by Occult study (clairvoyant), which distinguishes "ultimate physical atoms" by their direction of motion, the ever-spiral force moving from right to left in the positive, and from left to right in the negative; the former pouring out force and the latter receiving it (see Bibliography).

There are as many grades, shades, and hues, of color as of musical tones and combinations of geometrical forms; so the further we go from the so-called primaries of red, yellow, and blue, the more intricate, baffling and mysterious are these color relations.

Blue has been called the *negative* in nature which holds all things. Now, replacing "blue" with *indigo* we have an Occult truth. From the earliest ages Eastern philosophers have associated indigo with the spiritual, or higher mind of man (the Causal Body) ; but the curious properties of indigo have always been as well known to the practical dyer as to the Occultist. It is lighter than any known liquid and as long as it retains its color and nature it is insoluble even in ether. Therefore, the dyer must extract the blue by means of deoxidation.

In this process, called "setting the blue-vat," indigo gives us a perfect object lesson of the transformation in a substance according to its negative or positive conditions. When being made soluble indigo loses its *apparent* color in proportion as the oxygen departs, becoming perfectly white in solution. Goods dipped in the white liquid are then hung in the air, when they swiftly turn blue as the indigo in them is oxidized. Repeated immersion in the blue-vat gives every shade of blue from "sky" to "navy." As long as dyeing remained an art (until commercialized by the introduction of analine dyes), indigo was considered the only real blue dye (the woad of Gaul and Britain was a northern indigo and acted similarly) ; and with red, yellow, and brown, furnished the dyer with the natural substances from which he could make all the shades, tints, and hues his art required.

As you know that the earth vibration, *Prithivi,*

is yellow, it is of interest in this study of the *Tattvas* to add one bit more of dyer's lore. Herbs which yield yellow dyes are the commonest ones in forest and field. They were called by our forefathers, "greening weeds," because green was obtained by dyeing the stuff first in the indigo-vat, and then greening it to the desired shade in yellow dye. Now, just as *Âkâsha* is the omnipresent *Tattva*, synthesizing all others, so indigo corresponds with *Âkâsha* not merely symbolically, but because it is *Âkâshic* — a *Prithivic* form of *Âkâsha* — and holds other colors in synthesis.

You understand that the seven colors of the solar spectrum — so-called prismatic colors — distinguish the seven Logoi one from another; hence they are emanations from and manifest the characteristics of the Seven Hierarchies of Being, "each of which," says Mme. Blavatsky, "has a direct bearing upon and relation to one of the human Principles, since each of these Hierarchies is, in fact, the creator and source of the corresponding Principle." This statement confirms all the planetary correspondences and influences explained in earlier chapters.

As every Hierarchy is itself septenary, containing the seven colors of the spectrum, the permutations in colors are myriad, but the ruling or distinguishing color of a Hierarchy gives the hue to that septenary, for its influence is paramount. This is the primary source of all the *Tattvic* permutations and comminglings. To this infinite gamut of color in the realm of Nature the solar spectrum itself bears witness, for long ago, Sir David Brewster succeeded in counting not seven only but 2,000 Frauenhoefer lines which registered as many distinct tints and hues of color. Only the *Tattvic* Law can explain these as visualizing the varied geometrical forms of etheric vibrations. The seven prismatic colors correspond to simple, or primary forms; and their infinite variations to permutations of these.

As of everything throughout the Kosmos, there is septenary division and progression of races; and, as is quite generally understood, we are the Fifth Sub-race of the Fifth Root-race. We are in the Fourth round of this evolutionary cycle; that is, our globe is at the lowest arc of the planetary chain, the deepest involution of spirit in matter, and the period of the fullest development of pure intellect; a conbination that has produced the gross materialist,— the intellectual giant *sans* soul. But it is of profound significance that we are far past the *middle* of the round. Thus all is preparing for the Fifth round in which matter will lose its density. Why? Because faculties will be developed that enable man to perceive the withinness of all things. In Occultism, "There is no 'above' as no 'below,' but an eternal 'within,'

within two other withins, or planes of subjectivity merging gradually into that of terrestrial objectivity,—this being for *man* the last one, his own plane."

Just as every thought has form and consequently color, so sounds which, you know, are differentiated one from another by *form*, have their distinguishing colors, hues, and tints. Speech, which is sound in this physical world, *echoes as color* in the astral sphere around us and has its influence. All the wonderful harmony of color that delights our eyes has its correspondence with an inaudible harmony of sounds. The entrancing colors of nature,—the blue dome of the sky, the violet and purple of distant mountain heights, the green cadences of forest and meadow, the gold of the sunlit fields of ripening grain, the red of the igneous rocks and the fresh-turned earth,—all these are the visible tones of the "Harmony of the Sphere."

"The totality of the Seven Rays," says Mme. Blavatsky, "spread through the Solar system, constitute, so to say, the physical *Upádhi* [basis] of the *Ether of Science.*" To the seventh sense these inaudible sounds will be as perceptible as are the colors of musical tones to the clairvoyant now. The rudiments of the sense of sound exist in the minutest fragments of the Universe. The subtle space-granules — *Sûkchma-Âkâsha* — are everywhere, sound is inherent in them, not to be dissociated from them; but the sound varies, as you know, according to the form of the vibrations moving through this all-pervading space. It enwraps and penetrates even the minutest conceivable atom in the proportion of being greatly in excess of that atom; and color attends and irradiates this marvellous world of activity.

The perfected man who has evolved these higher senses — and woe to him if he misuse them; his fall will be abysmal — comes into possession of seven soul-senses, so to speak, corresponding with the physical senses but as much finer and more subtle in their vibratory force as the soul is higher than the body. It is these spiritual senses that will carry us beyond gross matter. The soul-senses corresponding with the sixth and seventh are the ability to recognize true inspiration, and the capacity to know the truth of being; that is, to communicate with spiritual intelligences in the wordless spaces of *Chit-Âkâsha*, or spirit-space, which is the "knowledge-space" of Swâmi Vivekânanda.

Not words but color and thoughts communicate ideas on this plane, and their vibrations are of varying degrees of subtilty; for every plane follows the fundamental law of septenary unfoldment. It is a region of marvellous color; etheralized, luminous colors of exquisite rainbow hues, ripple and flow with inconceivable velocity, not to be compared to anything upon the physical plane. Here is the light that never was on sea or land. The invisible world is radiant with it.

Dr. Babbitt calls it: "Psychic light, the direct messenger and servant of the spirit in its relations to the outward world." He further affirms that these psychic colors " reveal the primary laws of force "; and it was upon these that he based his wonderful and successful system of color therapeutics (*Principles of Light and Color*). There are from eight to ten octaves of color in sunlight of which not quite *one* is visible to ordinary human eyes. But culture improves the range of even physical vision, as artistic training constantly gives proof.

Realize now, that man is compounded of all these forces, being an aggregation of atoms through varied combinations and permutations, forming a center of the highest activity, through and upon which these myriad forces play continually. These forces are therein further transformed and pass out as evil or beneficent influences, *according to the use man has made of them*, to find their affinity in other centers. Up to this point, though you have studied only the five-fold nature of the *Tattvas*, every opportunity has been seized to impress upon you that they are vehicles for a higher, directing and overruling force,— that they are differentiated forms of that one dual force. We have found correspondence of the *Tattvas* from *Prithivi* to *Âkâsha* with five of the human sheaths, but there are seven sheaths. The logical mind at once demands: Are there not then seven *Tattvas?*

Yes, or no, according to the definition we give the word. If we restrict it to " an elemental condition of matter," there are but five; if we adhere to our higher signification, " a form of motion," that is, force within substance, there are seven. In the Upanishads, emphasis is everywhere given to the " five elements," and when a sixth principle is mentioned, it is consciousness or understanding. If seven are enumerated, both of these faculties are included. Thus power of choosing and directing is always implied. In the *Dharma Shastra* this explicit statement is made: " With the minute particles of the five perishable elements, every existing thing has been formed in its sequence and order." Who or what is the Former? The highest Principle. This is a very clear distinction which should be kept in mind.

Intuitionally we know there must be seven forces corresponding with the seven sheaths; so we seek to identify the two upper sheaths with what the fine inner sense has foreseen,— the Omnipresent Spirit, Âtma, and its individualized ray, the human soul,— the forces behind all force, and penetrating all. Thus, the sixth and seventh *Tattvas* correspond to Buddhi and Âtma — soul and Spirit. The latter is described by Mme. Blavatsky as " the Auric Envelope impregnated with the light of Âtma."

Naturally, these two higher *Tattvas* are as concealed from the average mortal as are the sixth and seventh senses from the materialistic mind; for just as *Âkâsha* — the all-pervading ether of space — has become cognizable only to comparatively recent science, and is yet but half-understood, a baffling paradox, so men generally cannot yet grasp the power and significance of the higher Principles and the planes of consciousness to which they will lead.

Until shortly before she was taken from her work here, Mme. Blavatsky was not permitted to reveal any information concerning the *Tattvas*. The embargo was, however, removed in time for her to state some facts in the appendix to the third volume of the *Secret Doctrine*, where she gives the names and powers of the higher *Tattvas*. She explains: " The doctrine of the seven *Tattvas* (the principles of the Universe and also of man) was held in great sacredness and, therefore, secrecy in days of old, by the Brahmans, who have now almost forgotten the teachings. Yet it is taught to this day in the schools beyond the Himalayan Range."

The sixth *Tattva* is *Anupâdaka*, described as

"The first differentiation on the plane of being, or that which is born by transformation from something higher than itself." It is the first garment, or sheath, of the spirit, and the color is said to be yellow. This I believe is its positive phase, and that negatively it is violet, which identifies it with Mercury whose phases correspond. The seventh *Tattva* is *Âdi*, the primordial universal Force. It is the vehicle containing potentially all things — Spirit-substance, Force and Matter.

"In Esoteric Cosmogony," says Mme. Blavatsky, "it is the Force which we refer to as proceeding from the First or Unmanifested Logos — Spiritual substance." The Sanskrit meaning of the word is "first," and in the Upanishads, *Âdi* is described as "The first, *i. e., Om.*".

As nearly as we can comprehend in our present stage of evolution, this highest Principle is a ray, a spark from God's self, which permeates the entire being, radiating from center to circumference. This makes perfectly clear and realizable St. Paul's affirmation that "He be not far from every one of us: For in Him, we live and move and have our being."

This one out-going energy is differentiated in the sheath but *not in Itself*. It is the Will of God; and man's will, when controlled by wisdom and understanding, shares in this spiritual power. This is the conquest of the Argus of fate.

If you comprehend what this implies, you will be convinced beyond the possibility of forgetting, that Higher Manas — well named the Causal Body — has power to mould every cell, molecule, and atom in the lower sheaths to whatever measure of purity and harmony the soul may dictate. *Manas* is spiritual self-consciousness in itself, and Divine consciousness when united with Buddhi. But only through a spirit of aspiration and self-consecration to the highest can this union of *Âtma-Buddhi-Manas* be attained, and realize for us the full activity of the spirit.

You already realize that the physical self which you know best is a sensitive harp played upon by myriads of vibrating waves. The Principles, or sheaths, are the tones in the human octave; and the individual keynote is the tone and has the color of the Principle most highly developed. The self clearly proclaims itself, its stage of progress or evolution through the colors which permeate it through and through, and radiate in its enveloping aura.

CHAPTER XXIV

COLOR IN THE VISIBLE AND INVISIBLE WORLD

Part II

IT is important to understand very clearly what is the personal responsibility for the key to which the Self responds. When this is comprehended and kept in mind, the frequent objections to the public teaching of these Truths of Being — which hastens the evolution of the Soul as nothing else can — and the periodical alarm cries concerning the dangers attending the practice of Yoga breathing exercises will entirely cease, for they will be recognized as baseless, the utterance either of ignorance or misdirected caution; both of which retard the advancement of the race.

In a very learned work, *Phenomena in Spiritual Being,* translated from the Tamil by Sri Râmanâthan, it is stated: "Not until ' the day of the flesh '— the days during which love of sensuous enjoyment prevails — has completely passed will *Tirodhâna Shakti* [veiling power] manifest Itself as *Parâ Shakti*" [all-illumining power]. *But* it depends upon ourselves — upon our desires and the thoughts we permit to cherish and nourish these — how long " the day of the flesh " shall endure!

Further, 'tis said: " The Giver of all knowledge, the great Teacher of the Universe, therefore withholds knowledge till the time of maturity arrives "— Yes; but *we hasten or retard that time by every thought* and act! To know the responsibility is to know the penalty for disregarding it. Evasion is utterly impossible. Here is the safeguard against misuse of power.

In the Upanishads we read that the human body made by the gods (Sephiroth) is the divine lute; that made by man himself is an imitation of it. The fingers of the divine lute correspond with the strings of the man-made; and we tighten or loosen them, we tune them to harmony or leave them to jangle ourselves. Discords are self-made.

Remember that the individual key and color depend upon the predominant sheaths, or Principles. While the strongest influence upon this is the composition of the *Prânic* currents at the hour of birth (that is, the exact hue or tint of the Hierarchy ruling the moment; the *Tattvic state* of the currents in the Hierarchy and flowing thence determining this), you have learned that the dominant thoughts of the mind and the consequent activities of the life have an overwhelming influence in modifying and changing these. There is no evil which has not its opposite good, and every key can be transmuted into good. Misuse and ignorance create all evil.

Irritability in the temperament makes a scarlet cloud in the *Kâma rupa* (frequently alluded to as the astral body) which is the plane of vivid emotions and passions; and every outburst of temper suffuses the whole sheath. When the tempest of passion dies away, the color fades out, but ever leaves a little more, a larger cloud of the passion-taint; and all the atoms of that Principle are more susceptible to greater heat and excitement upon the next occasion of loss of self-control. All actions, both good and bad, are thus received by the various vehicles and reflected in them, changing the hue of the color from moment to moment; and thus man forms his habits and from them builds his character; live, sentient atoms, pulsing with his thought, being the bricks and mortar of his structure.

Very fortunately the Causal body rejects all evil, which stamps itself only upon the lower and less permanent sheaths, the matter of which has greater affinity for evil. All good and uplifting influences are steadily stored up in the Causal body, making it stronger and more powerful to overcome, and thus the evolution of the soul goes on in spite of man's waywardness.

So the tones and consequently the colors of the human lute are irrefutable manifestations of what the Self is making and moulding out of the opportunities of this life, for they indicate his varied states, physical, mental, and spiritual. Thus the tone- and color-body of man reflects the man himself as in a mirror. This is the unvarying law of color, which ever and always betrays the media through which it flows, and the substance whence it emanates. And according to the prevalent color of the individual is that individual played upon and affected by the color in the external world; for color produces sound and sound produces color, the interaction of the two being invariable.*

The quality of a Principle is, of course, conditioned by the elements which compose it, and these give it a distinguishing color. But the shade or hue — and character and disposition depend much upon this — is determined by the number of its atoms, not considered in multiple or quantity, but in grade from one to seven,— degrees of subtlety or density; for every Principle has its septenary divisions of *Tattvic* permutations, and this varies the order of the colors. The physiological effect of the excess or deficiency of the normal color of a Principle is profound, and every disturbance of a *Tattva* causes exactly such disorder.

The difference in the effect of such disturbance upon different persons brings out in strong relief

---

* For interesting physical experiments proving this law, see Mrs. Besant's *Building of the Kosmos*.

the planetary influences which determine temperament and characteristics; for every Principle, simply reflecting the power of its ruling Hierarchy and *Tattva*, which works always in the matter of that sheath, has its special seat of influence in the human body, and exactly according to the so-called " accidents of birth " (there is no " chance," all is the effect of a given cause), primarily is a man prone to disorders of the head or feet, the heart or lungs, the stomach or liver, etc. But all these so-called " heriditary " weaknesses can be overcome by healthful living and more healthful thinking; thought being preeminently the moulding power of evolution, as it was in the beginning of involution. Voltaire said, as the sum of forty years' searching for truth: "*Chance is a word void of sense. The world is arranged according to mathematical laws.*"

Every organ in the body is the center of a certain power, and it is upon the perfection of its function and the harmonious co-operation of all these powers, that the well-being and usefulness of the individual, his growth and development to high purpose, depends. We are held " Under the Law " (Karma) by evil, not by good. In the life of the spirit we are freed and make laws for ourselves. The purity of soul-vibrations — soul-power applied to the regeneration of the body — has power to expel many seemingly malignant disorders.

Color in the Visible and Invisible World 275

Two facts must ever be kept in mind: The duality in all existence,— manifested and unmanifested, — it is the coexistence of spirit-matter; and that all development proceeds primarily by the triadic process. According to the stage of the process, from the creation of a universe to the birth of a human being and the thoughts of his mind (upon which *his* evolution depends), the color corresponds with and indicates the period, in varying grades marking the "critical" state,— or merging together of positive and negative phases which produce secondary colors,— from red through yellow to blue. But, never forget, above these and penetrating and modifying all is a spiritual force, without which they could not exist, which emanates as violet and indigo, for these are its garments. This spirit-force, the lowest form of spirit, manifests on the material plane as electricity and magnetism, and is to be identified as a ray from "The Light of the Logos." *Âkâsha*, limiting its form, "introducing the principle of division into the one," says Mrs. Besant, "veils the *Light*, and by limiting the ray, makes separation, where, essentially, separation there is none."

It is these varying phases and *Tattvic* combinations in every Hierarchy, planet, element, and corresponding human principle, that account for the discrepancies in the many schemes of correspondences between planets, *Tattvas*, elements, and

Principles. The so-called "secondary" colors, which are "critical" states and triadic, are sometimes called "neutral points" in progression, but they also have their dual phases; thus violet which comes forth from the mingling of positive red with negative blue, is the negative "neutral," and yellow, which occupies the middle ground between red and blue, is the positive "neutral." These two colors represent the corresponding phases of Mercury, and they are preeminent in the aura of an Adept during the state of *Samâdhi* when the *Kundalini* has risen in the *Sushumnâ*. Violet really veils the heat and light of the spiritual flame, and derives its potency and delicacy from the exquisitely subtle refinement of this electric fire, which is beyond the comprehension of our finite senses.

It is ultra-violet, of course, to which this refers; but all violet is intrinsically the same in nature and in influence, though lowered in degree of power as it is coarsened in descent through lower octaves to visibility.

Mme. Blavatsky declares numbers in connection with Principles "are purely arbitrary, changing with every school. Some count three, some four, some six, and some seven." She further explains that they do not follow in regular sequence, and that every student is left by his Guru "to work out for himself the number appropriate to each of his Principles." In a certain sense this is true; yet there are correspondences of tone, color, and Principle which, however they may vary individually, are best comprehended by assuming a normal order.

If we hold in mind the fact that all evolution, all progression, is cyclic, or spiral, it will help to a clearer comprehension of some puzzling statements; for degree and number must depend upon the grade — the height on the spiral — of the color and key.

CHAPTER XXV

COLOR IN THE VISIBLE AND INVISIBLE WORLD

CONCLUSION

AS we have found order, law, and system throughout the Kosmos, there must be order, underlying Mme. Blavatsky's seeming denial of it, in the numbering of the human principles. Her statement is true in the sense that the vehicle most highly developed is the most prominent one in the individual, and its color overshadows all other.

Now, if we think of the predominant sheaths as representing the tonics of a scale, the septenary beginning with the Tonic, the C-scale man would number from his Tonic, C, and the F sharp man from F sharp, and color and Principle would vary correspondingly.

Among the repeated references to this variability of type changing the order of Principles, Mme. Blavatsky says: "The human principles elude enumeration because each man differs from every other, just as no two blades of grass on the earth are alike." She also says: "Every man being born under a certain planet, there will always be a predominance of that planet's color in him, because that principle will rule in him which has its origin in the Hierarchy in question."

The speech of man preserves the record of time-honored recognition of this fact. We say: "He has a martial bearing." "His is a fiery temperament." "She was always a little luny"—meaning not crazy at all, but fanciful, imaginative. The very word *lunatic*, however, expresses the baleful effects of the moon's excessive and malign influence. "Even as a child he had a lordly way." That is, Jupiterian, commanding. "A Saturnine disposition" has its happy contrast in a "sunny" one. And thus, "A man of iron," "She is as good as gold," "He has no sand,"—these all are significant of elemental constitution. Pages could be filled with examples of this graphic symbology which has enriched all languages; and remember that all symbology is the expression of facts and truths. In losing sight of this, the moderns have suffered much.

At first the mind refuses to accept this mere pre-eminence of a sheath as changing its relations in kind or quality to the other Principles; but it becomes possible when we realize, to use Mrs. Besant's words, that "the sheaths are not divisible one from another," and that "there are but three

Upâdhis in which these different principles work;" that is, considered as planes of consciousness correlating man with the astral and physical, the psychic and mental, and the upper triadic or spiritual realms. Thus the physical body and its Etheric double are connected with the right eye, the positive center of vision dominating the senses. The *Kâma-rupa* and Lower *Manas*, with the brain; and the higher triad, with the heart. The Occult signification of this is, that the Spirit — Âtma — establishes centers of union for these closely allied sheaths in these organs, and the development of consciousness in the various sheaths proceeds from these centers. But this must not be considered as contradicting the fact that there are seven states of consciousness. There is neither sameness nor monotony, but varying degrees everywhere.

Lack of order exists also in the sense that none of the sheaths are *above* or *below* one another, for they interpenetrate and intermingle. Thus there is really no higher nor lower, but an eternal withinness. An example from physics will explain this most clearly. A cubic-inch of water expands into a cubic-foot of steam. In a glass globe of a cubic-foot's capacity *filled with steam*, not only can boiling water be added but also alcohol which will expand into just as much vapor as if no steam were present. After this, as much ether may be poured into the globe as if the space were not already occupied by steam and alcohol-vapor. A familiar experiment with solids is to fill a bowl with peas, scatter over it mustard-seed or other fine grain to fill the vacant spaces, then add salt and sugar. Just in this manner the atoms of the various human sheaths, varied by conditions of vibrating form and color, mingle together.

Annie Besant says: "*Every sphere is around us*, the astral, the mental, the buddhic, the nirvanic, and worlds higher yet, the life of the supreme God; we need not stir to find them for they are here; but our dull unreceptivity shuts them out more effectively than millions of miles of mere space" (*Ancient Wisdom*). But granted all these irregularities and blendings one with another, there yet must be a standard correspondence of Principles with *Tattvas*, colors, tones, and numbers. To ignore it, is to lose sight of the profound influence and significance of number,— to forget that it was and is — through the rhythm of vibrations — an unchangeable factor, with unchanging relations to the Hierarchies and the Principles emanating therefrom, because numerical relation is inherent in form.

In the sense of progression from the coarse vibrations of the physical plane to the inconceivably subtle ones of the spiritual plane, we have a mental concept in which the numbers of the sheaths must be unvarying. When we deal with involution, we may begin with Âtma as one and count down to seven. But our immediate concern is with the evolution of the soul in its conquest of the realm of matter. We are seeking to develop its freedom and power, seeking to free our real selves from the tyranny of uncontrolled sheaths of matter, and necessarily we must begin with the lower or coarsest vehicles. Therefore, we should logically count from one upward to seven, and the lowest sheath should be the most completely dominant or perfected of the physical principles.

The "Path" now is a spiral progression upward and outward; involution was a descent downward and inward. Our task is to release this inward power, not *from*, but *through* its gross material vehicles, *that it may be active in all;* and we must seek it within. To do this we must understand the sheaths in which the power is involved. Therefore the important point is to know them by association with their corresponding centers of physical activity, which are invariable, and with their normal colors and their tones or sounds. We must learn the separate tones first before we can combine them into harmonious chords and evolve melodies.

Remember that the sounds are seen, not heard on the physical plane. Mme. Blavatsky cites *Exodus*, xx. 18., in support of this, and says, when correctly translated the passage would read: "And the people saw the Voices, and these Voices,

Color in the Visible and Invisible World 283

or Sounds, are the Sephiroth." Spiritual man corresponds with the higher circles, "the Divine Prism which emanates from the One Infinite White Circle; the ultra-octaves of color and tone; while physical man, "emanating from the Sephiroth," corresponds with the lower octave of visible color with "the objective sounds that are seen, not heard."

Want of agreement exists wherever many minds have attempted to formulate a *part* of this law of correspondences without bringing all into harmony. But this very failure is evidence of the infinite variety in the permutations of the *Tattvas* and their alternating phases — omnipresent duality — and of the varying hues that every thought imparts to the atoms transmitting that thought or created by it; as also of different stages of development of the clairvoyant who describes the colors of these thought-and-sound forms. A clairvoyant may be able to see lower sheaths in an aura and not the higher ones. The lesson to us is to ignore unimportant differences — differences which are yet mere matters of intellectual guessing — and confine our attention to the facts which affect life and happiness.

The scheme of correspondences I have prepared is offered tentatively, because no authority can be quoted for it as a whole, but after much study and thought and comparing all authorities, it is the only one evolved from the tangle of discrepancies which appeals to me as logical and rational. The fundamental correspondence must be that of vibrations, and upon the coarseness or fineness of these all associations must be based.

When we speak of coarseness in this connection, and especially in reference to color, it must be understood in a comparative sense. Thus, red vibrations, the largest waves of visible light, are so small that 39,000 of them grouped side by side cover only one inch of space. The agreement of red with the fundamental tone in music was early recognized, each being the coarsest vibration of its kind; and in the procession of octaves of both color and sound, it was found that the closest ratio of like progression existed between the Tonic chord, or first, third, and fifth, and the triad of colors, red, yellow, and blue. The earnest student of the *Tattvas* must already have perceived that this triad, predominating in the solar plexus, exercises a preeminent influence upon the functions of life.

Now, Nature has taken such care to prove the agreement between tone and color that she has not left us to depend solely upon the psychic vision of the clairvoyant who sees the colors of tones and voices, but through remarkable cases of sense abnormalities has furnished us with indisputable corroboration of these relations.

In Berlin an operation was performed upon a

man's brain which required the severing of both the auditory and the visual nerves. When the nerves were reunited they were mismated, the upper portions of the optic nerves being joined to the under sections of the auditory nerves, and *vice versa*. The result of this distressing blunder is that the man *sees* sounds and *hears* colors. Looking at a red object he heard a deep base tone, and when blue was shown, the *sound* was like the tinkle of electric bells. But the ringing of an electric call-bell produced the sensation of blue light, and listening to Beethoven's " Pastoral Symphony " caused a vision of green meadows and waving corn.

The celebrated Italian scientist, Professor Lombroso, had an " hysterical " patient who lost her eyesight completely, but was able to read with the *tip of her ear*. As a test, the rays of the sun were focused upon her ear through a lens, and they dazzled her as if turned upon normal eyes, causing a sensation of being blinded by unbearable light.

Still more puzzling to Professor Lombroso was the fact that her sense of taste was transferred to her knees, and that of smell to her toes. This abnormality is very simple to the knower of the *Tattvas*, who recognizes these locations as centers of great activity for the *Tattvas* corresponding with these senses; that is, *Âpas* in the knees, and *Prithivi* in the feet.

Corresponding with the above-mentioned triads

of color and of tone, there is a triad of form, the triangle, cube, and sphere, or circle; and the chemical elements recognized as most closely related to these triads are respectively hydrogen, carbon, and oxygen. But they are none of them simple *Tattvic* forms; that is, hydrogen, recognized by Babbitt as "the *champion heat atom* of the world," is a *Prithivic* form of *Tejas;* carbon, a *Prithivic-Prithivi;* and oxygen, a *Prithivic-Vâyu*. Mrs. Besant says the scientist has as yet discovered no atoms that are not of this physical or terrestrial form,— all are *Prithivic* states of matter. He has as yet no conception of the six "higher atoms that stretch beyond." But the scientific view of the atom is rapidly changing as we have before this had occasion to notice. Already it is recognized that the atom is a complex not simple unit. A single atom of radium contains 160,000 electrons or corpuscles!

Science is fast taking down the walls between the visible and invisible, and ere another decade is marked off on the spiral of Time the materialist will be recognized as the true degenerate. All atoms of recognized chemical elements — so-called — admit of *four* dissociations, or separations, to simpler, more subtle states before the "ultimate atom" is reached. Students, who are interested to pursue the subject farther are advised to study Annie Besant's *Occult Chemistry;* and the work of Dr. Babbitt, previously mentioned.

With regard to the ether (*Âkâsha*) which pervades all space, science has at last come to this very rational conclusion, as Robert Kennedy Duncan puts it: "How much we ourselves are matter and how much ether is, in these days, a very moot question" (*The New Knowledge*). Science has discovered also that absolute immobility — rest — is non-existent; that every particle, every atom of the most solid-seeming matter is in an incessant quiver, and *that the velocity of the motion is constantly changing*. Is not this corroboration of the *Tattvic* Law, which alone can explain the phenomenon?

Think not that these details are a digression from our subject. They are, on the contrary, intimately connected therewith; for it is most important as a preparation for understanding the subtle sheaths of the body that the reader's imagination be wonted to faring forth into this marvellous world of the infinitesimally small, a clear conception of which is so much more difficult to form than of the vastness of the Universe.

CHAPTER XXVI

THE NORMAL COLORS OF MAN'S PRINCIPLES

Part I

NO problem of Occult knowledge has excited more controversy than the one we must now consider,— the correspondence of the Principles with color and tone, and therefore with number. For myself, I think it not merely unwise but impossible to surround it with hard and fast lines. To suggest the reasonable scheme — the one that imagination can accept, and in things Occult it is of paramount importance to see with the imagination — is the utmost I shall attempt.

There is deep insight as well as truth in the statement that " those who receive the wisdom of the past or the impressions of the present as something to have and to hold, gain absolutely nothing." That is, one must form *original* mental concepts of everything; receive all light, all suggestions, with open mind, but think, ever *think, oneself,* till more light is thrown upon the subject. The very nomenclature employed in this subject, the multiplicity of names for a single sheath, betrays the

The Normal Colors of Man's Principles

difficulty experienced in defining and accurately limiting the activities and influences of the separate Principles.

To guard against the possible misunderstanding that these correspondences can be defined with narrow dogmatism, I shall try to ensure a broad outlook, inviting individual thought and opinion, by giving the student first a glimpse through the mental eyes of Mrs. Besant and of Râma Prasâd.

The former says, " It is written in the *Mundâkopanishad* that from Brahman the One . . . comes Life — *Prâna* is the word used. I shall show you presently that *Prâna* is *Atma* in outgoing activity; the mind, *Manas*, that is the second; then the five elements as we know them — ether, air, fire, water, and earth; seven in all. These are the seven regions of the Universe, the seven sheaths of Brahman, as the SELF of the All " (*The Self and its Sheaths*).

As you already know, man's sheaths correspond with these and put him in touch with the entire Universe. Mrs. Besant's is a very simple classification, and clearly indicates the specific *Tattvic* action in the five lower sheaths, but she follows them in descent from three to seven, instead of ascent.

Râma Prasâd looks at the subject differently but is equally clear. He gives the human Principles as First, *Sthula Sharira* (gross body); second, unhappy *Prâna;* third, unhappy mind; fourth, happy *Prâna;* fifth, happy mind; sixth, the Soul; seventh, the Spirit (*Nature's Finer Forces*).

Thus he places *Kâma* — unhappy *Prâna* — and Lower *Manas* next the visible body over which their uncontrolled desires have so unhappy influence. These sheaths are those builders of Karma that have so potent influence in retarding evolution. Happy *Prâna* comes next Higher *Manas,* or the Causal body, these being the sheaths through the development of which the soul is released from bondage to the lower Principles and attains the power to bring them into sympathetic unison with her own higher vibrations. Remember that the Causal body is the chief agent in evolution, and is so called because in it are gathered the effects of experiences, which " act as *causes,* moulding future lives." But all the sheaths have their use in the economy of nature. Only their misuse renders them " unhappy."

Notice here that the fundamental five-fold division of body, life (the subtle-sheath), mind, soul, and spirit, corresponding with the five lower *Tattvas* which you know best, is expanded into the septenary by including the two phases of life — as vitality exhibited in actions — and of mind,— the thoughts prompting the actions and determining whether they shall be evil or good.

The scheme is somewhat misleading, however,

for *Prâna, per se*, cannot be restricted to number and sheath since it is the *Life in every sheath*. Mme. Blavatsky gave emphasis to this fact, and though she gave *Prâna* a number in some diagrams, she omitted it in others. In many classifications it is included, generally as the third Principle; but the lowest plane of *Prâna* is compounded of the microbes of science. "Fiery lives" direct the constructive work of the building microbes. The co-ordinating power of all these sheaths lies in *Prâna*. It is through *Prâna*, by means of the nervous system that the "I," the personality of the body, acts upon and through them all; and is responsible for the development of individuality as Desire yields to the direction of Will, and soul-force becomes an active and determining principle in the life.

In all schemes of correspondence there is one unvarying agreement,— the relation of Mars to the fire-element *Tejas*, and to red and the *Kâmic* sheath, or desire body; but in number it is variously considered as first, third, and even fourth. As the body of living fire within, the *Tejas* sheath seems essentially the first, for without it life would be impossible. The lowering of normal temperature is the first cause of most disease. The preponderating influence of desires in moulding the physical form, emotions changing the expression of the face even from moment to moment, and the thoughts that prompt them building character hour by hour, is sufficient reason for assigning to this sheath the lowest place in the evolutionary spiral. Of this sheath Mme. Blavatsky says, "It is the grossest [that is the coarsest] of all our Principles." The expansive character of *Tejas* vibrations and their vapor-like nature, give them this marvellous permeating and moulding power which enables them to enwrap the solid, cohesive atoms of *Prithivi* and become visible as red, and audible as Do, or Middle C, the Tonic of the first major scale.

The lower the race, the more visible is the color of this sheath, but more of this when we study the aura. *Kâmic* atoms are diffused throughout the blood, but are specially active in pelvis, liver, heart, and lungs. The whole trunk of the body, including the shoulders and arms, is greatly influenced by *Tejas*, and there are also subtle connections of this sheath with the left ear and the little finger of the right hand. The liver is the general and the spleen is the *aide-de-camp*. All the work which the liver shirks falls upon the spleen. This accounts for the fact that when a man's liver misbehaves, he is very apt to be "spleeny"; a most trying condition due to the fact that his spleen (that supposedly *superfluous* organ!) is overworked.

During the life of the physical body, *Kâma* is pronounced "a shapeless thing," but after death its astral atoms form a separate and distinct entity, which strives to attach itself to the Higher Ego. Mrs. Besant, *(The Seven Principles of Man,* p. 20), makes the nice distinction of confining the use of the term *rupa* (Sanskrit for " form ") to this after-death " vesture of animal nature," which exists in the astral sphere for a length of time proportioned to the tenacity of the physical desires which created it.* Being devoid of ethical sense, possessing only the lower animal consciousness, its rapid disintegration is the greatest blessing. Thus *Kâma* is the most material Principle in the human septenary group, hence the sheath whose composite links of desires for material pleasures and experiences bind us fastest to the physical plane and retard the Soul's progress.

The second Principle is the *Sthula-sharira* (gross body), corresponding to *Prithivi* (earth) through its state of matter, solid; but in color and tone, because so permeated by *Tejas,* with orange and Re. It influences the nose, lower posterior lobes of cerebrum, the liver, and the lower limbs from knees downward. Orange has always been recognized as synonymous with physical force; and it is, perhaps, for this reason and also as

* It is possible that Mrs. Besant does not hold this opinion now; for in a later work, *Ancient Wisdom,* she distinctly says that as the astral body [*Kâmic* sheath] develops, "it assumes the likeness of its owner * * * a body fit and ready to function and able to maintain itself apart from the physical." (Pp. 98-9.)

being the color of the gross body, that Occultists assign this color to vital-force, or *Prâna*. This, however, is not the teaching of the *Shivâgama*. Râma Prasâd, who follows the Sanskrit work, describes the positive current of *Prâna* as "reddish-white," and the negative, as "pure white; both being modified and tinged by the flow of the *Tattva* at the time prevailing. This teaching is corroborated by known physiological distinctions between the sensory and motor nerves; the former — the receptive and negative — being bluish-white; and the latter — the outgoing, positive agents — reddish gray. The Tantrists always refer to the negative, or *Rayi* as "the cooler state of life-matter, which is only a shade of *Prâna*, the original state." *Rayi* receives the impressions from "the motion-imparting phase of life-matter," — that is, the positive phase of *Prâna*.

Yellow is the color of the purest state of *Prithivi*, the spiritual element in the earth, its ensouled force, and predominating in the solar-terrestrial currents flowing round it; therefore, it is uncommon in the crust of the earth, which is composed of the grossest of its manifold permutations, but shines forth in its perfected things — the most precious metal, the citron fruits, ripened grains, and flowers. The fragrance of flowers is a spiritual essence stimulating to the nerves and conveying direct nutriment to the soul. Yellow is a very precious color, deemed the culmination of light. I think it could be proved that the foods most valuable to mankind are yellow. The liver is most favorably affected by oranges and by herbs of a yellow or orange hue, which are also cerebral and nerve stimulants; vitalizing, therefore, to the whole system, and laxative. The more harmonious the human body becomes and the purer and higher the aims of its indwelling Soul, the stronger, more electric and magnetic is the flow of the *Prithivic* currents through the *Nâdis*.

The *Sûkshma-sharira*, or Etheric-double, third Principle, is under the rule of Venus; for it corresponds with *Âpas* (water), and in color and tone with yellow and Mi. But, being composed of four grades of subtle ethers, the red and the blue Principles are present to form its negative violet. The absorbent, solvent, and reflecting powers (as in a mirror!) of this *Tattva*, and therefore of the sheath, whose substance has like qualities, make it inadvisable to attempt to establish hard and fast color-rules in their connection. Holding the septenary of colors latent, receiving colors from every source, and reflecting everything above and below, who can say positively that *Âpas* is this or that? In its primary state we know it as *white* and colorless. But we *can* venture to assign it an orderly place in the scale of progression as the normal state after permutations fitting it for physical activities. The moon is sometimes designated as the ruling planet of this sheath; but are not *all negative* conditions influenced by the moon? I believe it will eventually be proved that they are. Violet is the color sometimes attributed to the moon — a marvellously translucent silvery violet, the hue that silver assumes in certain conditions — and her mysterious power over water has always baffled the scientist. There are no doubt very subtle and strong relations between the moon and Venus.

The spleens are the vital links between the gross and etheric bodies, for through them *Prâna* is brought forth upon the physical plane. The subtle spleen absorbs the vital currents and transmutes and changes them into the coarser particles that become in the gross body its " elemental lives," animating the molecules and cells. The positive connection of these *shariras,* through motor nerves, is within the *medulla oblongata;* and the negative union, through the nerves of sensation, is in the solar plexus. Brown-Séquard says, " When a violent sudden emotion causes death, it is by the action on the *medulla oblongata."* The explanation is that the shock ruptures the union of the physical body with its double and thereby severs connection with the vital force (see Chapter XXII). The thoughtful reader will recall in this connection the prevalence of *Âpas* — stimulator of taste — in the throat.

Besides these profoundly important centers, the little finger of the left hand is influenced by the Etheric-double (through the spleen, as is the right through the liver; the little fingers corresponding with these organs), and it is this sheath which transmits all sense perceptions to the *Kâma-rupa*, the sheath of feeling and sensation; hence, in the Etheric-double lies the mysterious power to receive them in abnormal ways, as seeing through the ears and smelling with the toes. By so much as one sense is weakened or dulled is the connection between the Etheric body and its counterpart impaired.

One immediate benefit derived from practicing the breathing exercise for *Prânâyâma*, or control of *Prâna* — the exercise distinguished as the "Held Breath" — is that it invigorates and harmonizes all these immensely important connections, restoring them when disordered to their normal balance and union, and by so much as they are strengthened, strengthens the hold upon life itself.

The psychic breath is the breath of the spirit, and we cannot limit it to the thought-power setting into vibration the molecules of the nerve-cells. It is also the subtle breath of the Etheric body through the pores of the skin and it is something altogether finer than oxygen and nitrogen that it inhales in this psychic breath. The purity and healthful activity of the skin thus yields in importance to no other function of life.

CHAPTER XXVII

THE NORMAL COLORS OF MAN'S PRINCIPLES

CONCLUSION

SINCE *Prâna* is the unifying and vitalizing force between all the Principles, its special vehicle, the Etheric body, is subtly related to all, though most closely permeating, in the form of vapor, visible to psychic sight as a perfect shadow, the physical body of which it is both prototype and counterpart; for not only does it foreshadow coming disorders, but also it preserves in its etherealized copy the mark of every wound or blemish even after they are effaced from the physical body. No surgeon's knife can sever the limbs of the Etheric body, and it is this sheath that preserves the sensations of an amputated leg or arm. Iamblichas defined this Principle as " an unchangeable body of light which does not need anything for its sustenance." It is the *evestrum* of Paracelsus. Every life has such a body.

The healthful, normal activity of this Principle is of immense importance, for it is the medium through which the higher Principles of the human constitution penetrate the lower ones, and are ever trying to elevate them. This effort, arising in Buddhi, is man's conscience.

All anaesthetics, narcotics, and nerve tonics disturb the connections and the flow of the *Prânic* currents between these two *shariras*, affecting first the brain connections which become partially paralyzed. The resulting low vitality of the visible body is due to this separation from its prototype; the double, half-withdrawing from the left side, where psychic vision *sees it* as a violet-gray shadow.

Lower *Manas* is the fourth Principle and *Vâyu* sheath, under the rule of Jupiter; and it corresponds with two colors and tones according to the influence to which it yields. It is so prone to be ruled by desires that it is often called *Kâma-Manas*, and in this positive state it takes the complementary color of *Kâma*, green, with the tone Fa. When aspiring, and therefore receptive to vibrations from Higher *Manas*, it reflects blue with the tone Sol. This Principle is the thinking power of the physical man (the objective mind), functioning in the brain and nervous system. Through opportunity or ambition, a man may acquire marked intellectual ability without possessing even a dawning sense of the powers of Higher *Manas*. This is the condition of materialists, who may be strong personalities without gaining individuality, being complacently satisfied with the tremendous development of the lower self.

This sheath influences the *corpora-quadrigemina*, — another mark of its pronounced duality, the right ear, and "throat or navel," says Mme. Blavatsky; that is, blue vibrations above and green below.

Manas Antakarana — which corresponds with the pituitary body — is the imaginary line of communication between Higher and Lower *Manas*, — between personality and individuality; that is, it is the base of the triangle or the upper line of the square forming the lower quaternary according as we view it. The battlefield of life is in this Lower *Manasic* sheath, where desires wrestle with Thought for empire over the Self. You know how the elevation of this thought power develops Will, and uniting with it wins the victory for good. No fact is truer or of more vital significance than that " everywhere man *is* what he *thinks.*"

Higher *Manas*, the fifth Principle, is the *Âkâsha* sheath, ruled by Saturn; and corresponds with indigo and the tone La. Its physical seats of influence are the pituitary body, pineal gland, and the head as a whole. Activity in the pineal gland leads to the union of Buddhi-*Manas*. Psychic vision is stimulated in the pituitary body, which is the organ of the psychic plane. By the exercise of free will, and all development of *Will* is a development of Higher *Manas*, it has a spiritual influence in the heart. When Lower *Manas* is completely under the sway of *Kâma*, or is absorbed in materialism, Higher *Manas* has little opportunity to betray the fact that it is the vehicle of immortal Truth and Wisdom. It is this Higher Ego whose development Yoga practices encourage. All flashes of intuition, all inspirational conceptions which father inventions, manifestations of pure genius,— these come from Higher *Manas*, which as "part of the Essence of Universal Mind," has access to all planes of knowledge and power, and *knows* independently of the brain's reasoning.

Buddhi, the Soul, vehicle of Spirit, is the sixth Principle. Its *Tattva* is *Anupâdaki;* planet, Mercury; tone Si; colors, violet in positive phase and yellow in negative. Its physical seats of influence are the pineal gland, right eye, a plexus between the shoulders, and the heart; and its spiritual influence is in the *Sushumnâ*. The spiritual earth-force is closely related to Buddhi, and its connection with the subtle body is recognized by the colors of the latter which are a lower octave and reversed in activities as are all things reflected upon the physical plane of illusion.

You know the seventh Principle as *Âtma*, or Spirit, and also as the Auric Envelope, or Egg. Its subtle *Tattva*, *Âdi*, forming the Auric Envelope, not merely envelopes but *penetrates the whole body,* and its source is a " Spiritual Sun " of which our sun is a physical reflection, or more probably the vehicle. It manifests as white, or blue of such transcendent delicacy and illumination as only those who have seen the play of inner colors can conceive. Of course this Principle synthesizes all colors as it does all tones, and therefore all the other sheaths.

The rationality of this classification will be best understood, if the student draw a square beneath a triangle and place the sheaths on the lines in the following order: At the base of the square, *Kâma, Tejas* (write color and tone also); left side, *Sthula-sharira, Prithivi;* right side *Sûkshma-sharira, Âpas;* upper line (and base of triangle), Lower *Manas, Vâyu,* with green below line and blue above; left side of triangle, Higher *Manas, Âkâsha;* opposite side, Buddhi, *Anupâdaki;* apex, *Âtma, Âdi.*

Notice particularly that this succession preserves perfectly the interrelations and paramount influence of sheath upon sheath as reflections, shadows, or rays one from another; and therefore does no violence to our previous conceptions of *Tattvic* activities, being reconciled to them.

With the yellow sheath above moulding its permanent form, and the red below thrilling it with its incitements to activity and emotion, it is most clearly demonstrable that the gross body corresponds with orange. The "states of matter" of these seven Principles from one upward correspond closely with fluid or vapor, solid, liquid, gas, ether, Psychic Force, or magnetism; and Spirit, or electricity.

Bear in mind that a fundamental difference in these sheaths is the character of the vibrations which, proceeding from the lowest to the highest are increasingly subtle and ethereal in the nature of their atomic particles. The highest cannot act directly upon the lowest. The medium of gradually increasing density is indispensable; and only as we purify and refine the lower physical sheaths do we fit them, through making them responsive, for manifestation of the real individuality — the Higher Ego and the spiritually alive soul.

The objective form is the only thing that is perishable; the ideal form lives forever. May we not draw the right and hopeful lesson from this fact? We have it in our power to work constantly for betterment to improve our ideal forms; and, by so much as we succeed, to externalize that betterment in our objective physical forms, which are the models of future ideal forms. This is the law of evolution, the law by which the atom is evolved to purer states and to higher power, developing the latent and potential energies, the wisdom and understanding to which our race is marching onward.

Every thought vibrates on the subtle mental plane first, then passes through the astral to the etheric before it rouses vibrations upon the physical plane, in the gray matter of the brain. Thoughts are things, entities, because the fivefold powers of the mind as already developed in our race, are all *Tattvic* powers of exactly the potency represented by the senses they respectively stimulate; and thus they unitedly impart sound, feeling, form, color, taste, and odor to the thoughts born of their activity (form and color are properties of vision, hence *Tejas* activities).

It is psychic force working through the mental plane which acts in all overcoming of physical disorder or weakness. It has power when properly directed to build up and invigorate the lower sheaths, restoring all to harmonious co-operation in the complicated functions of the perfect human being. Keep this in mind, too: In this so wonderful structure, when we speak of superiority or subordination — of one sheath to another — the statement is merely relative. *Every sheath is so important* in the perfection of its office that it yields nothing to another. They are all mediums of activity *putting the Soul in touch* with the experiences through which it evolves to the consciousness of its vast inheritance. Trials and sorrows are often necessary experiences to rouse the Soul from inertia, selfishness, weakness, or other wrong doing. *None of the sheaths are independent. All are different.* Harmony is incomplete without every note in the scale.

The Soul atom is mingled with other lower atoms but *never combined.* To understand this clearly, fixing upon your mind a clear picture of the law, let me explain a fact the chemist knows well: Oxygen in pure air is *mixed, not combined* with nitrogen. When these two gases are combined, according to the proportions used, the result is one of five deadly poisons. Now, this is exactly the internal process; that is, within the human entity. When the atoms of the various sheaths are mingled harmoniously, the result is physical well-being; when discord ruptures the rhythm of their vibrations and their harmonious (that is, *normal)* balance, disintegration sets in; the molecules are broken up, the atoms are variously combined, and disease results. It is the use or abuse of everything which makes for good or evil.

The substance of all Souls is the negative phase of Spirit; very literally, indeed, the garment which clothes it. Faith and aspiration are needed for the growth of the Soul, and we must bring the mind up to unison with the Soul. By the regular practice of meditation and concentration, that control of the mind is gained which inclines it habitually to those Kosmic influences which are antagonistic to all evil tendencies in the lower sheaths that check our evolutionary progress. " Faith," says Râma Prasâd, " is nothing more than a mental lucidity in which the yet unknown truths of Nature begin to throw their shadows forward. The mind begins, as it were, to *feel* truth in any and every place; and, drawn by the taste of bliss *(Ânanda)*, proceeds with greater zeal to work out the process of its evolution."

The macrocosmic psychic center which is the prototype of man's sixth Principle — Buddhi — " is the great reservoir of every actual force in the Universe." Therefore, " by contemplation of the sixth Principle of the Universe, a sympathy is naturally established between it and the human soul. Only that sympathy is necessary for the universal *Tattvic* law to work with greater effect. The human soul begins to be cleansed of the dust of the world, and in its turn affects the mind in a similar way; and therein the Yogi becomes conscious of this influence by the slackening of the fetters forged by *Prakriti* [matter], and a daily, hourly strengthening of heavenward aspirations.

" The human soul then begins to become a center of power for its own little universe, just as *Ishvara* [the macrocosmic Soul] is the center of power in His Universe. . . . When perfection is attained, all the mental and physiological *Tattvas* of the microcosm, and to a certain extent of the surrounding world, become the slaves of the soul " *(Nature's Finer Forces)*.

Thus it is that when we cease to fear her, Nature becomes even more than our friend and ally.

CHAPTER XXVIII

THE AURIC ENVELOPE. ITS CONSTITUTION

WHEN we talk about the Auric Envelope, which encloses the physical body in "a luminous ovoid mist," within and upon which the colors of the aura play, we are not describing something which is conjectured as possible or probable, but something which has been seen by many eyes. Although to the large majority of people it is invisible, except under extraordinary and exceptional circumstances, all persons of refined and sensitive perceptions are conscious of a distinction in the atmosphere surrounding different persons. The presence of one is always calming; of another, often exciting when not irritating; the cheerful person radiates happiness and courage upon all; while others are more chilling than a wet blanket, and the impressions received are as varying as the persons receiving them.

This marked something which differentiates our fellows one from another is their personal atmosphere which forms the Auric Envelope extending from some inches to several feet around every human being. That the silent invisible world about us is luminous with the refined colors of the subtle ethers whose vibrations are streaming through and surrounding us, playing upon us ceaselessly, is a fact the proofs of which accumulate daily. When our sixth sense is developed, we shall all see these, and the color-sensitives, here and there — psychically developed persons who are phenomenal now and who see these colors — are merely *avant coureurs* of the evolution to which our race is marching onwards. In growing more spiritual — and evolution must lead to this, it is the immutable Law — humanity will see through everything, making clairvoyance normal. The X- and N-rays foreshadow this condition when dense matter will be, so to say, non-existent, because man will perceive the withinness of all things.

It is a familiar fact to many now that the colors vibrating in this invisible human aura betray beyond all question to psychic vision the nature of the life lived; for the aura is formed by subtle emanations from the Principles most active in the body, the vibrations of which radiate from its surface. When clairvoyance is universal, every man will stand unveiled in character before his fellows; for every thought, passion, and emotion is registered in his aura in unmistakable colors, and the seeing eye even now knows the man for what he is. There will then be no need for courts and judge and jury. Guilt will proclaim itself and stand confessed before those it has wronged.

Science is anticipating this era when Truth shall stand unveiled (and incidentally preparing the minds of men to receive that Truth graciously instead of doubting the testimony of their own eyes) through the invention of instruments of wondrous delicacy that ingeniously enact the role of Grand Inquisitor, but without putting any screws on defy man to conceal the nature of his thoughts, whether he be guilty or innocent, angry or calm, melancholy or gay, studious or idle. And all this, note well, is achieved through registering the vibrating currents of the *unspoken thought* as well as of the speech of the subject.

Moreover, that these thoughts take body and form as they are sent forth, is proved by Dr. Baraduc's clever use of the camera. He has seized upon the photographic plate the exact form of these invisible emanations radiating from the human being. Dr. Baraduc calls his photographs "Portraits of the Soul"; but it were better to recognize them as indisputable, permanent pictures of *all the activities* of the human subject, whether they be on the lowest physical plane or aspirations of the soul. It is a most important service that these photographs fully establish by material proof the fact that every thought has its distinctive form.

That the rays from the human being are further

endowed with the mysterious power of radio-activity was proved nearly five years ago when Professor Goodspeed, of Philadelphia, made photographs in an absolutely dark room by rays from his own hands. You will remember that the discovery of radio-activity is the factor which within a decade has swept from under the scientist's feet most of the firm ground, the "fixed facts," of nineteenth-century science.

So, little by little, science is penetrating this invisible world of force; and every discovery but corroborates the Occultist's statements concerning these varying planes of consciousness whence every force emanates. The scientist is coming nearer and nearer to the *Tattvic* Law which underlies all phenomena. But it is most difficult for him to recognize that the external forces which act upon man — as the "waves" of light and of sound which stimulate sense perceptions — are themselves in turn acted upon,—that the thoughts, emotions, and passions of man are so many vibratory "waves" of physical or mental force going out *from him to affect something somewhere!* For every thought arranges astral matter in definite forms, the *soul* of the form being the thought.

It is inevitable that we all are limited in what we see by the media (our own auras) through which we must ever look out. Our judgment, our opinions, must ever be tinged by these media, transparent films of vari-colored vibrations, oscillating with inconceivable velocity; thus the vision of many people is very literally a " seeing through the glass darkly." Let us have confidence always in happy eyes, since their vision must ever be the clearest, looking out as they do through pure, harmonious, and refined emanations.

A very delicate, trained psychic sight is required in order to distinguish accurately — hence with authority — the various emanations in the human aura; but it is no uncommon thing now to be able to see the coarser vibrations of the lower sheaths and the five ribbon-like bands of Tattvic colors (from *Ákâsha* to *Prithivi*) forming a layer next the skin, in which the geometrical forms of the vibrations flowing at the moment can be distinguished. These are beautifully and clearly described by Dr. Marques in his *Human Aura*.

Only as the clairvoyant develops personally the Lower *Manasic* and Causal principles, is the psychic power gained to see the auras of these higher sheaths, for they are increasingly subtle and are alone visible to like refinement of consciousness. As psychic vision penetrates plane after plane, it is as if veil after veil were removed.

It is the desire aura, or emanations from the *Kâmic* sheath, which extends from ten to twelve inches outside the physical body, with which the lowest grade of psychic sight is most familiar.

This is referred to as the "Astral Body" by Mr. Leadbeater *(Man Visible and Invisible)*, and as it is composed of astral matter it is an astral body. But the intangible self that travels far from the body during life is the *Mâyâvi-rûpa*, or "illusion form."

According to Mme. Blavatsky, "The *Mâyâvi Rûpa* is composed of the astral body as *Upâdhi* [base], the guiding intelligence of the heart, and the attributes and qualities from the Auric Envelope" *(Secret Doctrine*, Vol. III, p. 560). It is created by the intense thought of the person, and on occasions has been done unconsciously. Only Adepts have the power to project this form at will, and they can endow it with strength and impart to it every appearance of tangibility.

Unfortunately, the term astral body has been used very loosely. But instead of any disagreement or controversy as to *which*, the Etheric double or the *Kâmic* sheath should be thus named, it were better far to understand that there are *different* astral bodies,— that the term is not specific. Mrs. Besant says: "Any body formed of astral matter is an astral body, but its properties will vary with the principles with which it is informed." The astral body is said to be molecular, however etherealized it may be.

The astral world is the next one in refinement of matter to the physical world which normal sight cognizes. The separation, like the different sheaths of our bodies, is one of condition not of place.

The septenary law holds good on every plane, and astral matter is of varying grades of density. There are, so to speak, astral solids, liquids, gases, and ethers as on the physical plane we know best, but all are finer. There is practically no limit to the subdivisions of matter by ever-increasing refinement of its atoms; and life is more highly vitalized, and form is ever more and more *plastic* as decreasing density presents less resistance to the thought-forces which continually change and remould it.

Ethereal matter is astral, and the latter name was given because of the luminous or starlike brilliancy of its most refined states. The matter of the lowest subdivision of the astral world, corresponding to our physical, scarce deserves the name, but wanting a better distinction we must use it. To astral sight the astral world is visible; but to denizens of that plane there exist the same limits of condition as here, self-created through the mental activities which in selecting the materials used erect the wall of separation.

The fineness or coarseness of the *Kâmic* astral body depends upon the emotions and thoughts that play through it during this physical life. In low states of development, desire, stimulated from without,— living entirely in external things,— rules both body and mind. Such persons are weak-willed, and are at the beck and call of every suggestion and impulse. They build strong *Kâmic* sheaths which furnish the plasma for enduring *Kâma-rûpas* of the grossest astral matter, — the most permanent astral body.

As the person increases in intelligence, if the *ethical keeps pace with the mental* development, self-control is gained and the activities of the life are prompted from within; thus finer materials are attracted, and the *Kâmic* sheath increases in size, becoming purer and more distinct and stable. The vibrations of all Principles gain in refinement and purity when the mind governs desires instead of responding to the outward stimuli of the senses, and only then can evolution proceed apace. It is the difference in the state of matter which raises all bars of incomprehension and misunderstanding. As we refine the vibrations of our different Principles we refine their constituent matter, and open to ourselves plane after plane of consciousness.

Remember, always, that the separation between these worlds, or planes of consciousness, is one of constitution, not of place. Encircling spheres are constantly alluded to, but they are "concentric, interpenetrating spheres." There is really no separation except of condition,— a fact constantly proved in concentration, when consciousness passes successively through these sheaths, withdrawing, as the state of *Samâdhi* approaches, more and more remotely from the purely physical to the highest spiritual.

The Psychic, or Lower *Manasic*, sheath grows exactly in proportion as the mind develops. With the growth of the higher capacities of the mind, the aura becomes a very beautiful, irradiating one, penetrating and extending beyond the *Kâmic* sheath. The all-pervading *Âkâsha* is the medium, or atmosphere, in which the emanations of the several sheaths flow and intermingle; while *Âtma* is both within and without, the force behind force in every vibration. Enveloping all, though limited by the self-development of the individual, even *Âtma* is constrained by the medium, its density or rarity, through which it manifests.

Thus the aura is an absolute revelation of the divinity within. When it emanates from a radiant center nourished by a spiritually alive soul, it proclaims the purity and light within by the greater size of the separate auras, and by the transcendent radiance of the colors.

CHAPTER XXIX

THE AURIC ENVELOPE: HOW AFFECTED

ALTHOUGH personal character determines certain prevalent and more or less permanent colors, the human aura expands and varies in colors and hues according to the nature and the intensity of man's thoughts and emotions, every thought having its effect. Thus the aura reflects absolutely what is transpiring within. Indeed, Occultists say, "The astral man, whose color is determined by his evolutionary progress, is the real man." The clearness of the thought-form depends upon the thinking; if one is vivid, so will the other be; and the purity and beauty of the colors depends upon the purity and virtue of the thought. Indefinite thoughts make forms as cloudy and vague as the forces whence they emanate. In such cases, the colors blend indistinctly. The dreamer to "dream true" must picture clearly. No effect is greater than its cause.

Of all psychic conditions no other is so infectious as depression, which grays all colors till indigo absorbs them. Worry, anxiety, and irritation also degrade the colors; vicious passions and vices pollute them. All degradation of colors by graying and browning changes and lowers their signification and coarsens their atomic structure. In every color this change is the seal of intense egoism, and usually of absorption in things material, in sordid and selfish interests.

Remember that Nature works the same on all her planes. God placed in her hands the implement of vibratory Force, and through the varied character of these vibrations she chisels all forms, making fine forces visible through their color which proclaims their character and effect. We have the reflection of all the "Forty-nine Fires" within us. It is a comforting thought that the possibility of every color, every hue, every tone — *therefore of all perfection — is within.* Verily a bewilderingly complex creature is man.

It is this variety of color which makes possible such a range of vocal power — especially influenced by *Âpas*, the water vibration — for every modulation of tone is the effect of a distinctive modification of form through *Tattvic* permutations; and hence has its special shade, tint, or hue of color. Different *tints* are produced by mingling a color with white; *shades*, by darkening or deepening with indigo or black; and *hues*, by the blending of color with color, which gives us green-blues, yellow-greens, and reddish-blues. Râma

Prasâd says, "Various diseases may be cured, and good and bad tendencies imprinted on the *Prâna* by the power of sound;" because sound imparts to the vital force its own colors, modified only in degree by the individual *Prâna* upon which susceptibility depends. Do you realize when listening to music that every tone has its distinguishing color and throws the ether and the air into vibrations of exquisite form, and thereby affects for good or ill the hearer?

Thus, a *Tejas*-colored song rouses heat and excitement (as witness the effect of all patriotic songs), and may provoke intense emotion. The *Âkâsha*-colored song deepens melancholy and may cause fear and forgetfulness; and as every emotion of the human heart has its color, the sound of that color tends to rouse its corresponding emotion. The important science of color therapeutics, or chromopathy is based upon this fact, as also all musical therapeutics, or "medical music" as the cult was called when *first revived* a hundred years ago.

The part that sound plays in our lives is so depreciated, so profoundly misunderstood, that too great emphasis cannot be given to these particulars; and repetition must be pardoned, for some minds can be reached only by such reiteration.

Here is a good maxim to be given a prominent place in the home:

Sound is ever creating something. Shall it be evil or good?

A few years ago, when the National Society of Musical Therapeutics was formed in New York, the newspapers took the usual lively interest in developing a "sensation," and interviewed many prominent physicians to obtain "views" on the subject. The ignorance developed was amazing. One of the most noted nerve-specialists (?) in town said: "I have found music attractive to idiots, degenerates, and persons of abnormal temperaments; but I do not regard it as a therapeutic agent. . . . A sonata of Beethoven's may benefit a lunatic, but in that case so would the rattle of elevated railroad trains." Thus this so learned specialist is unable to distinguish between building and disintegrating sounds — between harmony and disrupturing discord — and is absolutely deaf and blind to their corresponding effects upon the nerves,— man's sound-register!

Every tone of the human voice, whether in speech or song, shares with the thought it expresses in the effect upon the vital currents and their emanations in the auras. It affects instantly the aura of the speaker, then influences those of his hearers. Therefore is the training of the speaking voice of highest importance in the perfecting of the individual. "If the words we utter bear the color of the *Agni Tattva* [*Tejas*] — anger, love, lust —

our *Prâna* is colored red, and this redness turns upon ourselves. It may burn up our substance, we may look lean and lank, we may have ten thousand other diseases. Terrible retribution of angry words! If our words are full of divine love and adoration, kindness and morality, words which give pleasure and satisfaction to whosoever hears them — the colors of the *Prithivi* and the Âpas — we become loving and beloved, adoring and adored, kind and moral, pleasing and pleased, satisfying and ever satisfied " (*Nature's Finer Forces*).

As I quote the above, there is brought to my attention a most interesting result from experiments in chick-breeding in a great hennery which is conducted strictly upon psychological principles. From the hour the eggs (over 400) are placed in the incubator, the same attendant cares for them, turning and cooling them; and as he handles the eggs, he *talks to them,* telling them the germ of life is there, they must be good little chicks, and will come out of their shells in so many days, whatever it be. Like clock-work, on the twenty-first day, every chick peeps forth from its shell; and here is the point that bears upon our study: If the attendant be changed and a strange voice greet these just-hatched babies, they are panic-stricken and flee about wildly for refuge; but the *voice that has talked to them through the shell* for twenty-one days, *has power to reassure them* and restore confidence. Hearing it, every baby-chick turns toward the voice, begins to " cheep " happily, and to pick up food.

The hens in this model hennery are played to — violin music — on wet and gloomy days to keep up their spirits; and the record of egg-laying proves that it is an effective stimulant. It is wellknown that hens are greatly frightened by disturbing noises, the barking of dogs, thunder, fireworks, and other explosives. Is not want of care in this respect a fruitful source of the many failures in chicken-raising?

When told that the color of a tone affects the nerves, hold in mind the fact that color and sound are the visible and audible effects of particular energies. It is the vibration which produces the given effect, whether it be our eyes or our ears which receive it and transmit it over our nerves; and the varied effects produced upon human beings by the same color or music are due to the modifications of individual idiosyncrasies,— the peculiar colors active within and hence pulsating throughout every person's aura. Nature's seal, determining the key, modifies the response to external stimulants.

While the ability to distinguish the varied colors in the auras of our fellows is still an exceptional gift, it is at the option of all to test the power of visible color to affect, favorably or unfavorably, the whole complex human being; that is, to act upon him physically as a stimulant or sedative of organic functions; and to affect him mentally and spiritually as well.

The benefit derived from surrounding yourself with a certain color or wearing it is, that the objective presence of the color aids greatly in visualizing it internally, and by thinking the color till it is vividly present to your mental consciousness, you connect yourself with the *Tattvic* currents of that color and draw them to you to furnish the right substance for subconscious activity, which you by this means consciously direct. Thus you actively accelerate the beneficent work of the needed *Tattvas;* and in this way, rightly applied, color becomes a powerful aid in mental therapeutics.

The colors most commonly seen in the so-called *Tattvic* aura (really a misnomer, because *all* is *Tattvic*) are, from the skin outward, luminous pearl-white, blue, violet, yellow, red; or in reversed order from the luminous band. But there are many variations, as, orange-yellow, bright line, blue, orange-yellow, and red; or dark line (indigo?), red, yellow, blue, and lavender-violet, and these changes in order and in colors are of course indicative of characteristic activities. With every change of *Tattvic* and *Prânic* currents the intensity of the colors varies; the physical condition of vitality or fatigue is also plainly marked, and this whole chromatic band pulsates in rhythm with the breathing; broadening with expiration, and decreasing with inspiration. I think myself, though I have neither seen nor heard the fact conjectured, that this one phenomenon proves the "*Tattvic* aura" to be the psychic breath between the dense and subtle bodies (the *Sthula*-and *Sûkshma-shariras*).

The *Tattvic* currents split at the *pulse* and run up the fingers separately in the regular order, from thumb to little finger, of *Âkâsha, Vâyu, Tejas, Âpas* and *Prithivi*. The air (*Vâyu*) *Tattva* dominates the whole hand as the index-finger does its mates, and gives to it its remarkable tactile delicacy, its suppleness and dexterity. By examination of the pulse-vibrations and the finger auras, the Hindu physican discovers which *Tattva* is disordered and diagnoses the consequent disease accordingly. His index-finger is sensitive to any preponderance of "wind" in the body; his middle-finger (*Tejas*), to an excess of bile, and his ring-finger, to the condition of the phlegm.

Musical sounds affect the *Tattvic* aura, intensifying not so much the existing colors as their lines of conjunction,— the neutral point — and especially, the luminous band lying next the skin, which is mainly *Âkâshic*. This effect is not emotional, but indicates the inevitable mechanical, rhythmic connection of sound vibrations. I believe all crashing, tumultuous, warring noise causes a similar but greater disturbance, and that the irritating effect upon the nerves begins right here, the shock tangling the vibrations and even loosening the connection between the gross and subtle bodies. Emotional influences from music are much more powerful than these mere rhythmic disturbances in the color-changes induced throughout the aura.

The lower auras, *Tattvic,* Etheric double, and *Kâmic,* extend farther out in the order named, and follow in shape all the outlines of the dense body. The three highest auras have the ovoid outlines of the Auric Envelope; and the aura of Lower *Manas* —" intermediate in *form* as in *Nature* "— while ovoid follows the sinuosities of the visible body, especially the movements of the head and shoulders. The Etheric double has its own *Tattvic* aura reflecting faintly the colors and geometrical figures of that playing upon the surface of the dense body. Any physical disturbance which is immanent can be seen in this form-body, which is literally a shadow of the future. Thus, a lady, having a fair complexion, sat for her photograph and was amazed to see that her face in the negative was covered with specks. The next day she fell ill with small-pox! The camera had caught the Etheric-body.

It is in the *Kâmic* and the two *Manasic* auras that color plays most vividly and proclaims unmistakably the man within; for these are the desire and thought vehicles wherein the influences dominating and swaying the man set their seal of energy. The color is the outward indication of the force either used within, drawn by desire, or generated in *that mightiest engine for good or ill — a man's brain!*

Dr. Marques says: "Through the two *Manasic* auras expert observers can clearly see the fleeting impressions produced by the general thought-currents [universal prevalent opinions]; impressions which vary according to the receptivity of man's corresponding Principle." It is in the Lower *Manasic* aura that the psychic reads the past events in the life of the subject, for the negatives are all imprinted here.

I think it is a mistake to speak of these auras as emanations from the different sheaths; for I believe they are *the sheaths themselves,* all together making up *the aura,* and filling the Auric Envelope. Thus instead of many auras, we have simply the sheaths of the Principles composing the septenary man, showing in the aura exactly how they interblend; which Principle is most active, and how through increasing refinement of the component elements, the sheaths extend farther out, manifesting the same increasing subtlety of structure from within outward that we see in the physical body from *Prithivi,* in the bones, to *Vâyu* in the skin. If we hold this picture in mind, we have an exact correspondence in form and activities between man within his Auric Egg and the minutest atom. The earth, from its core to its outer atmosphere, furnishes a like correspondence.

The *Kâmic* sheath of the undeveloped man is a cloudy mass of dense coarse atoms, "fit to respond to all the stimuli connected with passions and appetites." Brickish-browns, hot inflaming reds, and murky greens are the predominant hues, with a trace of dingy yellow about the head. Mrs. Besant says *(Ancient Wisdom):* "There is no play of light or quickly changing flashes of colors through this astral body; but the various passions show themselves as heavy surges, or, when violent as flashes; thus sexual passion will send a wave of muddy crimson, rage a flash of lurid red. . . . The centers of the organs of sense are definitely marked, and are active when worked on from without, but in quiescence the life-streams are sluggish." At this stage, growth must come from outward stimuli, and often suffering, either physical or mental, is needed to rouse from a life of stupid inertia.

All good and unselfish emotions are steps in ethical and mental progress that improve this sheath by refining its constituent particles. Its outlines grow clearer and finer; characteristic colors begin to assert themselves as fixed factors; though changing, ebbing and rippling, under the impulse of consciously directed thoughts and activities. Sudden ecstasies of pure exalted affection fill the whole *Kâmic* sheath with whirling thought-forms of purest, luminous crimson, while a flush of translucent rose-color veils all the throbbing, pulsating hues beneath.

CHAPTER XXX

THE AURIC ENVELOPE: ITS COLORS

OF all the colors radiating throughout the aura, red and green have the most widely varying significations according to their purity or degradation. When these forces are uncontrolled they become "the red and green monsters within us."

Red being the lowest material vesture of the involved spirit was visible in the skin of the first of the seven races on our planet (we are the fifth). Though evolution has paled the ruddy tint from the exterior, it remains the color of pure flesh and blood; its vibrations furnish the heat which maintains the normal temperature of life; and it is the happy sign of health when it flushes cheeks and lips.

Under the present conditions of life — the average of racial development — exposure to sunlight is believed to be the principal factor affecting the complexion of people; black, brown, olive, and copper-hued races originating in tropic zones; and Occultists do not consider the color of the skin any criterion of the mental or spiritual state of the man within. Though he were white-skinned, the aura of a very vicious man will be a brown-red, or a hot black; the extreme antithesis of the dazzlingly luminous one surrounding an Adept, which " shines with a sun-like splendor far beyond all imagination in its glorious loveliness."

The Adept's Causal body is not only much larger than that of the less developed but its colors are differently arranged. Mr. Leadbeater says, " These no longer move in whirling clouds, but are in great concentric shells, yet penetrated everywhere by radiations of living light always pouring forth from him as a center. The order of the colors differs according to the type to which the Adept belongs, so that there are several well-marked varieties amid their glory."

Throughout the Auric Envelope of the perfected man, playing upon its luminous mist, can be seen " millions of tiny living geometrical figures of every conceivable shape, throbbing in incessant pulsations; and in the center of it can be distinguished in glowing ethereal colors the mysterious five-pointed double star, characteristic of Adeptship " (*Human Aura*, Marques). These geometrical figures, circles, crescents, stars, spheres, and triangles, are, of course, the *Tattvic* vibrations, and are a part of every aura, playing through every sheath; but are not so distinct in the aura of an ordinary person, becoming more and more visible as intelligence and especially spirituality develop.

All the gamut from the basest passion of supremely gross and selfish love to the most exalted affection can be traced in *red*. Absolutely unselfish love expresses itself in a lovely rose-color, and when it is exceptionally brilliant and tinged with violet, it indicates spiritual love of humanity and exalted maternal affection. Pure crimson denotes less elevated love; jealousy tinges it with brown, and selfishness mingles clouds of dull grayed green which sink below, while pride degrades it with orange. All heat and passion flush the aura with outbursts of red from the brilliant scarlet of righteous indignation to the lurid flame-color which cuts acutest triangular flashes through black hate-forms. Dark, dull red is passionate and earthy when not malevolent. After outbursts of intense anger, Mr. Leadbeater says, "Terrible thought-forms of hate may be seen floating like coils of heavy poisonous snakes in a man's aura."

The variety of green in the visible world is exactly typical of the versatile human characteristics which this color manifests. Its prevalence in the aura indicates strong personality, adaptability, and too often selfishness. But these traits may be high or low according to the shade and hue. Grayed and browned hues signify that shifting indecision which is all things to all men; really a selfish cowardice ever seeking its own ends, having evolved no principles beyond desiring the obvious advantage of the moment. This green abounds in the auras of those who permit others to do their thinking for them. Selfishness varies from brown-gray to bottle-green, and is, alas! very common in the desire sheath.

Green is preeminently a material color, and "greenbacks" are aptly tinted and named, for the financial currents of the earth are deep, bright grass green. Purely material phases of intellectuality, the brains that are absorbed in things external, cram with book-knowledge of the day, with statistics and crude facts, send forth vibrations of bright green.

Strong self-consciousness, the sense of personality, is vivid, clear green; and according to the striving for growth, the hope and aspiration felt, may shade from apple to emerald. Where soul-consciousness and *individuality* — as distinct from *personality* — develop, the green changes through peacock-blue to deep, luminous sapphire. Higher mental qualities which bring distinction in the arts and are nourished from springs of intuition vibrate in this exquisite azure.

All the music of the spheres vibrates in the indigo-blue of *Âkâsha*, in which are all colors and out of which they flow. With respect to music and other arts, Mme. Blavatsky says they are the children of either the Higher *Manasic* or *Kâma-*

Manasic principle proportionately as Soul or technicality predominates. Thus there will be more red and green in the aura of the technique devotee than blue. She further says: " Metaphysics are the domain of the Higher *Manas;* whereas Physics are that of *Kâma-Manas,* which does the thinking in Physical Science and on material things. . . . The Mathematician without spirituality, however great he may be, will not reach Metaphysics; but the Metaphysician will master the highest conceptions of Mathematics, and will apply them, without learning the latter."

Pure deep blue indicates devotion; pale sapphire, spiritual perception; and the light hues, as turquoise, cobalt, and robin's egg, exalted ideals and emotions. Yet blue, too, may be degraded. If grayed or muddied, the religious devotion is mere bigotry or selfish fear. Sudden fright casts a ghastly livid-gray veil over all.

It is almost superfluous to remind the student of the lofty character of yellow, or of its beneficial effects when prevalent in the aura. It spreads the joyous contagion of its own vitality, calming and stimulating at one and the same time as effectually as the gloomy, pernicious gray of depression exhausts and disturbs. So if you would benefit your fellows, see to it first of all that you radiate health-giving colors from your aura, which, you know, you cannot do unless you encourage the thoughts that create them. Not until the Causal body is developed sufficiently to control Lower *Manas* and *Kâma*, does this beneficent and forceful current find a favorable medium through which to act. The prevalence of clear, deep yellow and good pure green in the aura indicate a happy, generous, sympathetic, and hopeful character evolving to higher states.

Yellow manifests the highest and noblest intellectual effort, true wisdom and aspiration, freed from objective, material striving; and therefore represents the highest power and loftiest aspect of spirituality which our race is capable of grasping and understanding. The positive power of this Principle is proved by its dominance over all other colors with which it is blended. Pride vibrates as orange, but in the degree that the red is shaken out of it, is it raised to pure aspiration. Because of its penetrating power, yellow is the color most easily perceived by normal sight; and it has been visible as a veritable halo round the heads of speakers engaged in some supreme effort of enthusiasm which freed the soul to its fullest expression. In such cases the vigor of the astral vibrations rouses "a sympathetic vibration even in the coarse and heavy matter of the physical plane." Exalted spiritual vibrations cause a violet cloud to rise from the crown of the head in the midst of surrounding yellow of a luminous tint, and the violet sparkles through and through with golden specks.

It is in the aura of the pineal gland that perception is located. "This aura answers in vibrations to any impressions, but it can only be sensed, not perceived, in the living man. During the process of thought manifesting in consciousness, a constant vibration occurs in the light of this aura, and a clairvoyant looking at the brain of a living man may almost count, see with the spiritual eye, the seven scales, the seven shades of light, passing from the dullest to the brightest. You touch your hand; before you touch it the vibration is already in the aura of the pineal gland, and has its own shade of color. It is this aura which causes the wear and tear of the organ by the vibrations it sets up. . . .

"There are seven cavities in the brain which are quite empty during life. . . . These centers are, in Occultism, called the seven harmonies, the scale of the divine harmonies. They are filled with *Âkâsha,* each with its own color, according to the state of consciousness in which you are. The fourth is the pituitary body; the fifth is the third ventricle; the sixth is the pineal gland, which is hollow and empty during life; and the seventh is the whole. When *Manas* is united to *Âtma-Buddhi,* or when *Âtma-Buddhi* is centered in *Manas,* it acts in the three higher cavities, radiating, sending forth a halo of light, and this is visible in the case of a very holy person" (*Secret Doctrine*, Vol. III, pp. 577 and 583).

The front brain has a higher grade of colors than the back brain. The countless magnetic and electric curves which radiate from the head and surround it with a play of exquisite colors correspond vividly with the "Thousand-petalled Lotus" of the Yogi. The colors thus seen by psychic vision to emanate from different parts of the brain corroborate all that phrenology claims as to special seats of "faculties," or emotions and activities, and all that Occultists teach; and this statement holds also with regard to the whole body.

The heart is the center of spiritual consciousness as is the brain of intellectual; and all the play of light in the aura of the pineal gland is reflected in the heart's aura, "which vibrates and illumines the seven brains of the heart, just as does the aura round the pineal gland." Corroboratory of these statements is that of Dr. Babbitt that "The brain has been seen to have five great leading poles, or centers of luminous radiation, the greater of which is in the center, besides which it has minor poles in all the organs which connect with the center pole." Clairvoyants can see explosive flashes of light from all nerve ganglia, and wanting Occult training might fail to distinguish the septenary.

Although the colors of all these auras are as constantly shifting and changing as the waters in the seething whirlpool at Niagara, the particles pulsating with inconceivable velocity, yet yellow, rose, blue, and violet if present, are always found in the upper part of the aura about the head and shoulders; while red, from pure crimson to its hot, lurid hues, radiates midway, from shoulders to thighs; and the debased colors of debasing qualities are below. The purer the color the higher; thus most greens and deep orange are about the feet and lower limbs; but the pure green of versatility and sympathy is seen above the shoulders.

The all-penetrating, all-permeating force, binding all together, the aural light, is the manifestation of the Spirit within, which forms the "Envelope" or "Egg," and appears as a faintly luminous silver-blue-violet shadow, irradiated with the hue which gives the key to the individual. The more highly developed the person, the more distinct is this hue, the unmistakable mark of the ruling Hierarchy, and the evidence of the presence of the Special Ray connecting every individual soul with its Hierarchy.

Even a slight understanding of the nature of the influences with which men people the contiguous astral realm, influences which are constantly affecting man for good or ill, according to the nature of the thoughts and desires which he permits to dwell in his consciousness, would inevitably increase the sense of responsibility as to the purity and elevation of his habitual thoughts and aims.

Ignoble thoughts, selfish, jealous, or passionate thoughts, or the stings of deadly hatred, enter only the centers where like thoughts hold sway. So he who indulges such polluting, discordant thoughts draws added incentive to his own evil thinking, while heaping on fuel to that of his fellows. It is through the medium of astral matter that all our thoughts vibrate. They take form there instantly and change with the utmost rapidity, seeking always their affinity or pursuing the direction in which they are consciously sent. Every unselfish emotion purifies all the vibrations as pure air clears a smoky atmosphere. Loving thoughts help all the region through which they pass.

You see there are thought-forms just as there are tone- and voice-forms. Mrs. Besant puts this very strongly, and says thoughts may be angels or devils, and man is held responsible [not by a vengeful God but by Law] for their creation. And she gives this comforting thought: " Many a mother's loving prayers go to hover round her son as angel-forms, turning aside from him evil influences that perchance his own thoughts are attracting " (*Ancient Wisdom*, pp. 77-81).

Not only does all our real and lasting happiness here depend upon the use we make of our thought-power; but exactly in the proportion that we develop and gain control of the "mind-stuff" will be the perfection of that Heaven we all hope to attain after this earth-life. For Devachan, the heaven-plane, or world, is in substance *mind-stuff*, and it yields to us exactly what we have power to mould, to think into a reality; because every mental act takes immediate form there. Hence Heaven is as beautiful and perfect as we have the ability to make it.

The outflow of spiritual or psychic energy from the auras of those who through ceaseless aspiration are advancing rapidly on the Path is of marvellous potency. There is scarce a limit to be placed upon the beneficence of such characters, of the effect of their work and influence; their mere presence is felt as an inspiration, as a healing blessing. Aspiration is the exercise of the Soul, through which it grows to heights invisible. Who can doubt that the present awakening of the public conscience, the great moral wave sweeping round the world, is due to the pure vibrations emanating from the ever-increasing army of those who have come under the great Light through the widespread teaching of the Power of Thought to manipulate Life's Forces? It is the real "Life Science," explaining God's purpose and his Laws.

CHAPTER XXXI

HOW TO ACQUIRE RHYTHMIC BREATHING

THE whole Law of the Rhythmic Breath is now unfolded to you; you know its importance; you know that the vibrations surrounding every human being (as also *all living things* from plants upward) are exactly symptomatic of internal conditions, being outward manifestations of those conditions; and you must realize the importance of the character and purity of the invisible color-forces which compose the human aura. Therefore, there remains but to consider some details of the constant effect of the Law.

If we would hold ourselves receptive to the finer, purer *Tattvic* currents flowing about us, it is imperative that the irregular fleeting waves of color which commonly sweep rapidly as before gusts of wind through the aura, be reduced to regular rhythmic vibrations, otherwise they present a repellant wall. Given an earnest desire to improve, with control of those emotions generally recognized as evil, nothing else so degrades and lowers the colors as the all-too-common habit of depression; nothing else so purifies and refines them, and enlarges the aura, as the regular habit of deep, rhythmic breathing.

We must give a glance at some of the reasons for our having to learn carefully and slowly, what should be perfectly natural to every human being. The first function of life which is aborted and perverted is that of correct breathing, and no other function is so little understood or so ignored and abused. It is this perversion and abuse that sow the first seeds of weakness and disorder in the human frame, because preventing any possibility of the harmonically balanced rhythmic flow of vital-force.

The babe, before he has submitted to discipline's unnatural methods of development, breathes deeply, moving his abdomen more than his chest; because the diaphragm is superintending the normal function, and, when lowered, thrusts the viscera downward which distends the elastic muscles of the abdominal walls, and leaves the thorax above much enlarged for the full expansion of the lungs. Only thus can the lower lung-cells be filled or have their stagnant residue of air changed and renewed. Everything stagnant is impure and *invites germs of disease*.

The moment discipline treats the child as something that must be *bent* to civilization's standards instead of growing up naturally like a flower, constraint and fear begin their deadly work of tension and cramping, and nerves and muscles respond instantly to the iniquitous maldirection. Discord has set in and there is no more normal freedom. Fear clamps the lungs in a vice more harmful even than the external strictures of senseless clothing.

The long-suffering body, restored to its rights, and relegated to its true position in the septenary chain of human principles, becomes a totally different thing from the incubus which generations of men have dragged through life in the belief that ills of the flesh were the natural and unavoidable evils of living. Only the gross ignorance of the primest necessities of healthful living has created and fostered most of these ills,— an ignorance which in spite of a decade and a half of the most active propaganda to spread the cult of health and *prevention of disease through healthful living*, still blinds the majority of mankind; and to the neglect of no one prime need is so much suffering due as to deprivation of *fresh pure air!* The purer the air the purer are the *Tattvic* vibrations and the higher their potencies.

As life exists only from breath to breath, he who but half-breaths only half-lives; and reduces his tenure upon life to but a slender thread. The vital forces which are the source of all life and which maintain and renew it, enter our bodies with every breath; are rhythmic in the degree of its regularity, and their harmony and normal balance depend *first* upon *the freshness and purity of the air inhaled.* Every exhalation expels from the body noxious principles, wastes generated in the physiological chemistry of combustion processes, which are virulent poisons to *all living creatures.* Domestic animals and pet birds are even more susceptible to their deadly influence than is man himself, in whom unfortunately, the effects are slower and more subtle; else would mankind have awakened long ago to the loathsomeness of re-breathing these foul exhalations.

The cult of deep-breathing broke the first link in these self-forged shackles that mankind has dragged for so many weary centuries. But, unhappily, the cult was no sooner launched than it was split by theorists into many " schools " ; and according to the teacher the student was drilled in diaphragmatic, intercostal, or clavicular breathing; systems which divide the thorax into lower, middle, and upper registers respectively, and inhibit more than slight, imperfect movements of air through the practically unemployed cells of the lungs. It seems never to have occurred to these experimenters to ask (much less could they answer the query!) why so much space was taken up in the chest by masses of spongy substance that was of no use in the human economy, yet was so alarmingly susceptible to painful disorders!

It was never intended that only a part of the

lungs should be used, but men and women have each adopted their special method of defeating Nature; the former, from neglect of clavicular (upper chest) breathing, furnishing the more victims of tuberculosis; and the latter, from their constriction of the waist-line, inhibiting all the lower muscles from activity, thus often causing atrophy of the lower lobes of the lungs, and rendering practically immovable the vital organs just beneath the diaphragm; which encourages a long train of suffering. Semi-invalidism and early decay are inevitable under such conditions. Yet a New York authority upon voice-culture says that with correct deep-breathing, " no voice need lose its beauty till one, two, or even three, decades after the fortieth birthday is passed."

Now, deep, rhythmic breathing uses *no one* of these restricted " registers," but does employ *all three in one*. Habitual inhalations should be prolonged till every respiratory muscle has been called into action and every lung cell is distended. This cannot be accomplished without a *perfectly free* and strong elastic diaphragm. It is profoundly important that one learn not only how to make it so — faithful practice will do it — but also its exact office in this *life* function.

The diaphragm is nearly the shape of an inverted basin,— an irregular arch or crescent in every dimension. Acting like a bellows, when thrust *out* and *downward,* it expands the thorax, creating a vacuum into which the air is drawn, and it presses downward and outward all that is beneath it. Normal, deep breathing, which is rhythmic and harmonious, is thus an internal *massage* of all the vital organs. Every breath moves them gently in position, and consequently increases the circulation of the blood, and stimulates their secretions and excretions. The movements in both directions are partly contraction and partly expansion.

If you are not certain that your habitual breathing thus lowers and raises the diaphragm so the whole lungs are alternately filled and *emptied,* practice deep breathing while lying prone upon your back upon an unyielding surface. You will thus both *see* and *feel* the downward and outward stretching movement of the diaphragm as it flattens out when you *inhale;* for the abdomen is distended by the lowering of the viscera; and you will distinctly feel the pressure upon the small of the back where the diaphragm is connected with the spine just below the lowest rib. Its great anchoring muscles, there contracting, pull it down forcibly. This part should be distended as much as the abdomen, but at the beginning of practice is apt to be found inactive.

It is in the filling of these lower lung-cells that the favorable *Tattvas, Prithivi* and *Âpas,* put in their finest work of upbuilding and renewing. With every inhalation the abdomen should rise gently, falling with the exhalation, when the diaphragm is arched upward pressing upon and emptying the lower lung-cells.

When you have mastered the method, resume a sitting or standing posture for practice. In habitual breathing, the exhalations should be in rhythm with the inhalations, counting from six to eight during a movement according to lung-power, which will increase amazingly as the chest-walls and all muscles gain elasticity through regular practice.

The pulse — heart-beat — should be the unit of count, for the two functions are most closely associated. Thus: inhale during six pulse-throbs; hold breath during three; exhale during six counts; hold lungs empty during three counts. Repeat a dozen times or more; lengthen the breath as power is gained; and practice according to convenience several times a day. In normal, rhythmic breathing, the solar current flows *in* and *out* through the right nostril, and the lunar current through the left. When it is desired to make one or the other current flow, close the nostril or press the fifth rib on the side you wish to make inactive, and *inhale* and *exhale* through the other nostril. Inhale slowly and always through the nostrils, in which passages there is provision to arrest impurities which, if carried to the lungs, would irritate their delicate structure. Contagious diseases can be contracted by the unlovely as well as unclean habit of mouth-breathing.

Do nothing automatically. In all your practice, make your thoughts follow and direct the vital currents. For example: *Think* as well as feel the pressure and distention in the small of the back. You will thus greatly facilitate the forming of the habit of doing involuntarily what you must now practice. Moreover, indulgence in automatisms is dangerously apt to encourage absent-mindedness, a fault which leads to grave mistakes, the results of which are seldom confined to the immediate offenders. All the accidents due to the "Didn't-think" folk can be traced to the encouragement of automatisms.

The habit should be acquired of holding the breath perceptibly before the exhalation, for only thus do we take from the inhaled air all its vital elements. It is possible through faithful practice to wont ourselves to deep, rhythmic breathing as the rule; and with the help of the corrective exercises — Alternate Breathing and Held Breath — to develop a dynamic energy which we can divert at need to any organ or nerve of the body and hold there long enough to stimulate a revitalizing process.

When we gain control of *Prâna* — for which

purpose the Held-Breath exercises are practiced — we are able to feel its subtle activity all over the body, and can concentrate it wherever an exhausted nerve needs renewing energy. It is only in these corrective exercises, or when the need is felt to change the currents, that the nostrils are closed and the breath arbitrarily directed to left or right. When the balance of the alternating current is restored, we leave Nature to take care of their regular alternation.

Human beings are electric batteries; and when either current of vital force — the negative or positive — flows too long, the vehicle of life becomes the engine of destruction. That is all; it is just a simple problem of electro-chemical action; and the *Tattvic* Law is the only thing that explains the mystery by which human life hangs on so slight a thread, and indicates to you the remedy for time of need. The knowledge thus put in your hands is a treasure beyond price.

In all practice, the promptness of the body's response to the revivifying influence will be exactly according to the clearness with which you realize the thought and the fixity with which you can hold it. Directed consciously with your soul-force vitalizing your mental vibrations, the current of *Prâna* increases in strength and electrical power, so that all the atoms are drawn into synchronous action, which means enormously increased power and activity.

CHAPTER XXXII

THE PRACTICAL APPLICATION OF THESE LAWS

THE first application of the *Tattvic* Law is to realize that you are yourself responsible for the character of the forces active within. There is not an act of life nor a thought to which the Law does not apply; it expresses itself in the form of like vibrations everywhere and in everything. The forces of the Universe are playing upon and around you, and what you think and feel determines what sort shall find affinity within. But knowledge alone of the Law does not enable us to apply it,— does not give us the power to *use* the master key. That is gained only by steadfast determination and faithful practice of all means to the end. If one thing has been emphasized more than another in these lessons upon the Evolution of the Self through Health to Freedom and Power, it is the need of harmony from the foundation upward.

The perfect life — which can be made the common life *not* the exceptional one — permitting the unfolding of undreamed of powers of mind and soul, requires for its foundation a strong body whose equilibrium is maintained by the rhythmic functioning of all its complex organs, under the control of a sane, wholesome mind. Rid yourself right here and now of any belief you may have in the body itself being sinful. "Matter is not in itself evil. On the contrary, it comes forth from God, and consists of that whereof God's Self consists, Spirit. It *is* Spirit by the force of the Divine will subjected to conditions and limitations, and made externally cognizable" (*Perfect Way*, p. 41).

The whole end and aim of humanity's trials and experiences is to educate souls to overcome, to gain the Will-power "to escape the limitations of matter and return to the condition of pure Spirit." Remember the distinction I pointed out to you between the will at the beck and call of desire, and a Will which is the handmaid of Soul-consciousness and holds every thought under control. In the latter case only is the Will strong and really free.

To ignore the body and affirm that "mind is all," is both unscientific and a grave mistake; for while mind is ensheathed in the body all the vehicles through which consciousness manifests are efficient in proportion as their activities work together in rhythmic harmony for the good of all. Each must sound its own perfect note, just as the various organs of the body should; all together forming a harmonious chord. Only perfect health, with subordination of every organ to its legitimate function — as well-trained soldiers work together — permits the freedom and enjoyment of this condition.

"The aim of all endeavor," says Anna Kingsford, "should be to bring the body into subjection to, and harmony with the Spirit, by refining and subliming it; and so heightening its powers as to make it sensitive and responsive to all the motions of the Spirit." *The Law of the Rhythmic Breath* is the only explanation of Kosmic Forces which teaches how to "sublime" the body, and "make it sensitive and responsive" to the Spirit. A sound mind in a perfectly controlled body is indispensable for progress in the refinement and development of all the sheaths which leads to consciousness on all planes and to soul-knowledge.

As Annie Besant says: "All that is needed to be in Heaven [now] is to become conscious of those vibrations"; — that is, vibrations of soul-consciousness, higher states latent in all; but which require for their forth-coming conditions of peace, confidence, serenity, and poise. These are impossible in a pain-racked body, or in one heavy with the impurities of gross living and discordant thinking.

When the Spirit is deeply involved in matter (lower vibrations), inertia is manifested. We speak of being "heavy-hearted," "depressed in spirits," "sleepy," yet prolonged sleep brings no rest; *under such influences*, we are literally weighted down by the gross, heavy states of the physical atoms. As the Spirit, through the purification of matter, evolves out of it, the vibrations increase in refinement; and lightness, exhilaration, and elasticity are increasingly apparent. In such states we bring enthusiasm to bear upon all that we do, and every activity is a joy; work ceases to be labor. We have connected ourselves with higher and purer sources of energy.

Epictetus reminds us: "Men are distracted not by the things which happen but by their opinions about things." To consistently apply the *Tattvic* Law and reap the advantage from the knowledge of it which is possible for every earnest and determined soul, there is in most cases an imperative need to change the whole tenor of customary thought,— often, indeed, the order of the life; to purify the mind and body through wholesome thinking and living, with faith, charity, love, and truth, and effacement of all petty self-interests as the basis of daily activities.

The cheerfulness and joy resulting promote a state of harmony, for happiness, confidence, and courage are upbuilding forces; fear, anxiety, petty animosities, intolerance, resentment, and cowardice are *dis*integrating and *dis*cordant, because they *dis*-

turb the balance of the *Tattvas*, and greatly increase the preponderance of those which in excess are *dis*astrous. The physical and mental peril of indulgence in these latter emotions and thoughts, is not half-understood; but here, again, the *Tattvic* Law clearly explains cause and effect, warns of the danger, and places responsibility. We must learn to direct our activities and govern our lives systematically, refusing longer to be the playthings of chance. We must think clearly and plan our days so they shall be filled with the things worth the doing.

As a primary condition of peace, happiness, and health, you must rule your own forces. If you would attract harmonious conditions, your own mood must be harmonious and confident. When we recognize that we live in a world of forces of which *we are a part*, and that the soul-governed-and-directed will can control these forces, we realize our responsibility for the proper exercise of that control, through the right use and direction of the Power of Thought.

It seems the most stupendous blindness that men have gone on for centuries delving into this world of Effects — the earth and the life thereon — and persistently denied that the world of Cause could be anything outside of the unit under examination, — that they could dream of accurate results in studying one Unit of the macrocosm as an isolated world of Effect revolving upon itself.

Only the all-compelling Sun has forced man to recognize something of its influence; but so little does he comprehend it that he hesitates not to bar out its beneficent rays entirely from his dwelling, nor to build great factories and office-hives where thousands of helpless human workers are immured, delving by artificial light throughout the *Long Day!* Oh, the pity of it!

Since you know that the nature of certain thoughts must inevitably produce unfavorable vibrations, is it not as rank injustice to yourself and those affected by your mental or physical condition to indulge in them as it would be to take poison? As all vibrations can be controlled by thought, you must *think* the vibrations which you desire to be most active in your body. Not denial of pain and weakness, but conscious thought-construction of the conditions you would manifest in your life — just as the artist bodies forth on his canvas the picture his imagination has conceived — is the sure method to hasten the fulfillment of your strongest desires and aims. You *must* control your thoughts for they are always *creating* something. "The imaginative power in man is the reflection of the power that in God created the Universe" (*Evolution of Life and Form*, Annie Besant).

Râma Prasâd says: "As the balance of the

Tattvas brings comfort and enjoyment of life, so the sense of comfort and enjoyment which colors our *Prâna* and mind when we put ourselves in sympathy with the comfortable restores the balance of the *Tattvas*. And when the balance of the *Tattvas* is restored what remains? Disinclination to work, doubt, laziness and other feelings of that kind can no longer stand, and the result is the restoration of the mind to perfect calmness. . . . But, for such a result to be achieved there must be long and powerful application (*Nature's Finer Forces*).

See to it that you contribute no discord to your environment; if so unfortunate as to come in contact with it, be no party to it. By every act of your life set the example of poise, serenity, and happy confidence in ultimate good. Oppose passion and pessimism with *silent* thoughts of their opposites. There is much comfort in the knowledge that through beneficent suggestion we may often influence for good a nature which can hear no arguments nor opposing opinions without being stirred to excited antagonism. A mental atmosphere of love and confidence, protects us from all evil thought-waves.

It is necessary to give final emphasis to the fact that the exercises in Yoga breathing are not methods of regular, still less of rhythmic, breathing, but, as stated in the first chapter, are scientifically designed to restore the balance of the positive and negative currents which in normal breathing flow rhythmically and *alternately*, one *after* the other, at regular periods down the right and left sides of the spine; the right (positive) and left (negative) lungs being correspondingly charged. The excess of one current, or the undue preponderance of a *Tattva* causes *dis*order; then, if order be not restored, *disease*. It is the inception of *all* disease, organic as well as functional.

The normal order of God's vast Universe is based upon rhythmic harmony, and the healthful functioning of all his creatures upon this terrestrial globe is a reflection upon the gross, or visible, plane of activity of that perfect, harmonious rhythm. Mark well that I say *healthful functioning*. We all know that this normal condition is the blessing enjoyed by not more than one person in five hundred, if so many.

The present age not only suffers from many weaknesses resulting from the ignorance and wrong-doing of past generations, but has involved itself deeper and deeper in materialism, separating itself from the beneficent spiritual plane of its being, which has developed hitherto unknown diseases encroaching upon and impairing, more and more with the progress of this thing *mis-called civilization*, the channels of vital force, the nervous system.

The corrective exercises are designed to restore divine order, no function of life having been so misunderstood and neglected during centuries as the vital one of breathing. The difference between the two exercises is very great. They supplement each other. Alternate breathing renews and freshens the human battery, undoing the mischief created through having employed *one current* too long; it is nerve-calming and equalizing; for it restores the atoms to harmonious activity, when before they were all struggling for their individual " breath of life."

The Held-Breath describes itself, for though the breaths are taken alternately as in the other exercises, the *holding* is the important part. It is nerve-energizing to a greater degree — and acts more promptly — than any other remedy for nerve-exhaustion yet devised; because the thought, concentrating *Prâna* in different plexuses, polarizes the electro-chemical action, refines the *Tattvic* vibrations, and raises them to inconceivably higher power. This exercise for *Prânâyâma* (control of *Prâna*) thus electrifies all the nerves of the body and stimulates all the organic functions to their highest activity. I have had many proofs of its wonderfully purifying, renewing, and invigorating power when practiced regularly and faithfully.

Since we are human electric batteries, there is no slightest doubt in my mind that we can accomplish more for the regeneration of our bodies in this way — the force being infinitely finer — than can be done by the application of high-power currents from electrical machines. D'Arsonval's new apparatus (designed to destroy the "germs of old age") gives an alternating current of one thousand million vibrations per second. But the mind gains nothing by this treatment beyond having its house put in order *for it*. Without belittling that, I must remind you that the mind still remains the mischief-maker, which, uncontrolled, draws discordant vibrations that will quickly undo the good. Where the will-power is lacking to gain the necessary mental control, by all means try the electric-battery. That is the next best thing, but remember that it is only man's clever device to replace Divine methods, therefore incomplete.

This explanation amply refutes the charge that an "unnatural method of breathing is taught by Yoga exercises." Instead of "reversing the natural circulation of the blood, bringing abnormal pressure upon psychic centers in the brain," as one critic charges, the exercises, *if directions for practice be followed*, have none but the most beneficial and stimulating effect upon both the blood circulation and the circulation of *Prâna* (vital force) in the nerves.

Long experience has proved to me beyond the

shadow of a doubt that these corrective exercises successfully effect a purification and regulation of the Kosmic currents flowing over the nerves which, through restoring the normal balance of the vital-currents, restores harmony and consequently strength where heretofore discord and disease have held high carnival mainly because of the disordered and unnatural breathing which has become the rule among mankind instead of the exception.

Instances of harm resulting from Yoga exercises can always be traced to injudicious practice, because of ignorance of the forces used — the two phases of the vital-current and the *Tattvic* vibrations composing the currents. All wholesale condemnation and denunciation are based also upon ignorance, but are due to observed results of malpractice. Unfortunately, this very practice has been sanctioned and directed sometimes by those who command confidence because supposedly having been trained themselves in the oldest Eastern systems.

But I would caution you that no one who understands the *Science of Breath* would dream of instructing students to practice the Held-Breath exercise for long periods of thirty to forty-five minutes. The conditions thus produced *are* " unnatural " and destroy all normal activity. They are exactly what is described in the picturesque phraseology of the *Shivâgama* as the state when " the fires of death burn." The enthusiasts who thus attempt to develop psychic powers by a *tour de force*, to break into heaven, as they perhaps suppose, by scaling its walls, are hopelessly defeating any spiritual aspirations they may have. You cannot *burst* through the sheaths without shattering them; each must be refined in turn.

Again I say: Evolution is the reverse process of involution. We must begin with the body and its directing mind. Soul-consciousness is gained in no other way; and psychic powers are but a source of danger and tribulation, of weakness to the body and mind, until *both mental* sheaths are developed, the higher, sufficiently to recognize its power.

Here, again, Anna Kingsford indicates the *Perfect Way:* " It is vain to seek the inner chamber without first passing through the outer."

Concentration is not a practice to be restricted to the special periods devoted to it; but as facility and power are gained to hold the mind under control, the law of effective thinking and doing should be applied in all the affairs of life. It should become the fixed habit to concentrate the mind upon the affair of the moment no matter how trivial it may be. Only thus can the pernicious trick of mind-wandering be overcome; only thus can the mind be trained to efficient service at all times. And as it — the mind — is making you, hour by hour, what you are, is it not really the most important task in life to learn to direct its activities in ways beneficent instead of ways pernicious?

It is only when we can attain inward calm, can free ourselves from the tangle of the common daily perplexities and avocations, that we gain a true perspective of the things that so absorb us; realize the pettiness of most of them, separate the wheat from the tares; and cultivate a judgment that will successfully guide us and bring order and peace.

There can be no final word on this vast subject. Its profound importance has been made clear to all who are sufficiently interested to *think*. To such there will be no fruitless moments of thought and endeavor. Ever, as they seek, will the Path become more illuminated; and they and I must continue to learn as long as we strive for "More Light."

ENVOI

May God's blessing bring to every reader of this book enlightenment and ever-increasing understanding of Nature's Laws, which are inseparable from the Truth of Being.

GLOSSARY

The very name Sanskrit — abbreviated from Samskrita — implies the elaboration and subtle nicety of its structure, "the perfectly constructed speech dedicated to literary and religious purposes, but also the spoken language of cultured people"; and thus distinguished from the vernacular of the common people, Prakrita, or Prakrit, of which there are many dialects.

Although the Sanskrit alphabet contains forty-eight letters — thirteen vowels and thirty-five consonants — these are augmented by so many compound letters according as they are grouped in words, and to express shades of meaning and pronunciation, that about five hundred distinct types, or symbols, are necessary for the complete equipment of a Sanskrit font. The reason for this nice distinction is the conviction that number, form, and color are inherent in every sound.

Diacritical marks, corresponding somewhat to the Greek "breathings," under and over letters, both vowels and consonants, change their sound-value entirely; and as these lack significance to English eyes, having no correspondence with English usage, the best method to convey the pronunciation of Sanskrit words has been to spell them in English as nearly as possible phonetically. For example: the spelling *Sakti* gives no hint of the pronuncitation of the word. In Sanskrit the *S* would have a breathing mark over it by which the letter would be recognized as having very nearly the sound-value of *sh* in *shun*, or *ss* in *session*. Therefore, the spelling for the English reader should be *Shakti;* so also *Sushumnâ*, not *Susumnâ; Âkâsha*, not *Akasa; Shiva*, not *Siva*.

A is the most important vowel in Sanskrit, and its two sounds, long like *a* in *ah!* and short like *u* in *up*, are distinguished by a slight change in the letters. Short or "medial" a is considered inherent in every consonant, unless it is followed by another vowel. A typical word to illustrate pronunciation and common usage is *Pandit*, a learned Brahmin, which has become most familiar to English eyes as well as ears in the spelling *Pundit*, which preserves its pronunciation. In the English Theosophical works of the best-known writers, long *â* in Sanskrit words has the circumflex accent over it, and short *a* is without mark.

E has the sound of *a* in *may;* long *i*, of *i* in *machine;* short *i*, of *i* in *kin;* long *u* is like *oo* in *moon*, and short, like *u* in *push*.

Âdi — ah'dee; primordial universal Force. "The vehicle containing potentially everything."

Agni — ag'nee (*a* almost like *a* in *as*, *g* hard); fire, sacrificial fire, god of fire; name sometimes given to *Tejas Tattva*.

Âkâsha — ah-kah'shuh; subtle ether, fifth *Tattva*, the subtle sound-granules of space, without and within every atom.

Anupâdaka — on-oo-pah'du-ku; the sixth *Tattva*.

Amrita — om-ree'tuh; the nectar of the gods; the water of eternal life.

Apâna — up-ah'nuh; a manifestation of *Prâna*, down-breathing, eliminator of wastes.

Apas — ah'pus, a *Tattva*, water element, stimulator of taste, gustiferous ether.

Atma — aht'muh; the Spirit of the Universe, highest Principle in man.

Aum — ah-oo-mu (all blended together). The sacred word; its pronunciation needs to be heard; it may be pronounced as two, three, or seven syllables, setting up corresponding vibrations.

Avidyâ — uh-veed'yah; ignorance, darkness.

Buddhi — Bood'hi, understanding, wisdom, vehicle of the Spirit, connecting *Atma* with *Manas;* " the determinative faculty "; sixth Principle in man.

Chakra — chuk'ruh; a wheel, disc, a circling motion; a cycle of seasons or of years.

Chitta — chit-tuh; " mind stuff."

Fohat — Fo-hut; force in its highest, most subtle state.

Ghâri — gu-hah'ree (compound consonants like *ph, kh, th, gh,* and *bh* are aspirated separately as in *inkhorn, loghouse*); a period of twenty-four minutes.

Idâ — ee-dah; the negative *Nâdi* down left side of spine.

Ishvara — Eesh-wah-ru; the soul of the Universe, the same as Brahmâ, also the god Shiva.

Kâma — kah-muh; desire, longing, emotion.

Kârana-sharira — kah'ruh-nu–shuh-ree-ruh;   Causal body.

Karma — kur-muh; the moral law of compensation operating to produce all conditions of life; that force which operates to connect cause and effect unvaryingly.

Manas — mon-us; mind, the third Principle of the Universe from below.

Mantra — mun'truh, metrical word or verse having an essential rhythmic virtue; hence spell, charm, incantation.

Mâyâvi-rûpa — mah-yah'vee–roo-puh (see text for full definition); an astral body.

Mûla-prakriti — moo'luh–pruh-kree'tee; undifferentiated matter, from *mula*, root, and *prakriti*, matter, source.

Nâdi — nah'dee; a tube or a line along which something flows, applied indiscriminately to nerves, arteries, and veins.

Om, same as *Aum*, which see; "that undifferentiated word that has produced all manifestations."

Padma — pud-muh; the lotus, a center of nervous force.

Pingalâ — pin-guh-lah; the positive *Nâdi* on right side of spine.

Pradhâna — prud-hah'nuh; unevolved matter, manifestation of *Mûla-prakriti;* chief person or thing.

Prakrita — pruh-kree'tuh; the derived speech, the various East Indian dialects of the common people.

Prakriti — pruh-kree'tee; undifferentiated Kosmic matter. Nature.

Prâna — prah'nuh; breath of life, vital force, spirit, electricity and magnetism in different phases of the most subtle state.

Prithivî — prit-hi-vee'; a *Tattva*, the earth element, stimulator of smell, the odoriferous ether.

Pûrusha — poo'rus-huh; the personal life-giving principle in all things, human soul, Supreme Soul, spirit, the intelligence pervading Nature.

Râjah Yoga — Rah'juh Yo-guh; literally, Royal yoga, the conquering of the lower nature and uniting the soul with divinity, or attainment of soul-consciousness and realizing that divinity within.

Rayi — ruh-yee; negative phase of matter, lunar ray.

Samâdhi — su-mahd'hee; perfect concentration, a state of super-consciousness that carries one beyond the limits of reason; meditation bringing one "face to face with facts which no instinct or reason can ever know"; highest and last stage of yoga.

Samâna — su-mah'nuh; a manifestation of *Prâna*, on-breathing, active in assimilation and renewing processes.

Shakti — shuk'tee; the negative phase of any force; the seven *shaktis* correspond with the "sons of *Fohat*"; the consort of a god, the god being the *positive phase of a* force.

Shivâgama — Shee-vah'guh-muh; an ancient Sanskrit work attributed to Shiva.

Shloka — sh-lo'kuh; Vedic verses.

Sthula-sharira — st-hoo'luh-shu-ree-ruh; gross body.

Sûkshma-sharira — sook'shmuh; subtle or etheric body.

Svastika — swus-ti-kuh; a sacred symbol among ancient peoples of almost world-wide use; any lucky or auspicious object.

Tantra — tun-truh; Sanskrit treatises on the science of the human body and soul.

Tattva — tut-twuh; "the substance out of which the universe is formed," and "the power by which it is sustained"; the true elements; the essence or substance of anything; a form of vibration; truth, reality, opposed to what is fallacious. In compounds with other words, *tattva* always implies knowledge. In the original edition of *Nature's Finer Forces*, Râma Prasâd spelled the word *tatwa*, which gives the correct pronunciation; for although Sanskrit *v* has commonly the sound of *v* in *every* it is *softened* to *w* when *preceded* by a consonant.

It was sadly misleading, and has contributed much to the confusion concerning the pronunciation of this word, that the English editor of the later edition of Râma Prasâd's book changed the spelling to the Sanskrit form *tattva* without giving any explanation; and as all the other changes in orthography were to the end of indicating the correct pronunciation, the natural inference was that this came under the same rule. As a half-dozen dictionaries and as many Sanskrit grammars might be consulted without finding a hint of other pronunciation of *v* than in English *vine*, the above omission has tended to fasten this erroneous pronunciation upon the word. Monier-Williams' Sanskrit Dictionary gives the rule I have cited, and I have the further authority of a Hindu Sanskrit scholar for the pronunciation given.

Tejas — tay-jus; a *Tattva*, the fire element, stimulator of the sense of sight, the luminiferous ether.

Truti — troo-tee; a division of time, a measure of space; an atom; one hundred and fifty *trutis* equal one second.

Udâna — oo-da-nuh; a manifestation of *Prâna*, up-breathing.

Upâdhi — oo-pahd'hee; a basis of consciousness, of which there are three correlated to three regions of the Universe, sensuous, intellectual, and spiritual.

Upanishad — Oo-pun-ish-ud; ancient mystical writings, "secret knowledge."

Vâyu — Vah'you; a *Tattva,* air element, stimulator of the sense of touch and feeling, the tangiferous ether.

Vyâna — vy-ah'nuh; that manifestation of *Prâna* in which *Apas* is prevalent, all over the body.

Yoga — yo'guh; a division of Sankhya philosophy teaching methods by which complete union with Deity is attained (*yoga,* to yoke). The adjective descriptive of methods is also *yoga.*

Yogi — yo-gee (hard *g*); one trained in yoga methods; a contemplative saint.

BIBLIOGRAPHY

'Nature's Finer Forces. Râma Prasâd, M.A., F.T.S.
    (Theosophical Publishing Society, London and Paris.)

✗ *Râjah Yoga.* Swâmi Vikekânanda.
    (The Baker and Taylor Co., New York.)

Human Aura. A. Marques, S.D.
    (Mercury Office, San Francisco.)

Perfect Way. Anna Kingsford and Edward Maitland.
    (Theosophical Publishing Company, 244 Lexington Ave., New York.)

Principles of Light and Color. E. D. Babbitt.
    (Published by the author, New York, 1878.)

Secret Doctrine (3 volumes). Mme. H. P. Blavatsky.
    (Theosophical Pub. Society, 3 Langham Place, London, W.)

Isis Unveiled. Mme. H. P. Blavatsky.

Key to Theosophy. Mme. H. P. Blavatsky.

The Voice of the Silence. Mme. H. P. Blavatsky.

Upanishads. *Sacred Books of the East,* Vols. I and XV.
    (Oxford, at the Clarendon Press.)

Bhagavadgita, Sacred Books. Vol. VIII.

Buddhist Mahâyâna Sutras. Vol. XLIX.

The Vedanta Sutras. Vol. XXXIV.

The Laws of Manu. Vol. XXV.

Bibliography

Ancient Wisdom. Annie Besant.
Seven Principles of Man. Annie Besant.
Building of the Kosmos. Annie Besant.
Evolution of Life and Form. Annie Besant.
The Self and its Sheaths. Annie Besant.
Birth and Evolution of the Soul. Annie Besant.
Thought Power. Annie Besant.
   (Theosophical Pub. Society, Benares and London.)
Man Visible and Invisible. C. W. Leadbeater.
   (John Lane, London and New York.)
Human Aura. W. J. Colville.
   (Frederick Cole, New York.)
Auras and Colors. J. C. F. Grumbine.
   (The Order of the White Rose, Syracuse, N. Y.)
The Power of Silence. Horatio W. Dresser.
Education and the Philosophical Ideal. Horatio W. Dresser.
   (G. P. Putnam's Sons, New York and London.)
Phenomena of Spiritual Being. Translated from the Tamil, by Sri Râmanâthan.
   (*The Word,* October, 1904, to February, 1906.)
The Zodiac. H. W. Percival.
   (*The Word,* beginning in April, 1906.)
Influence of the Stars. Rosa Baughan.
   (Published in London.)
The New Knowledge. Robert Kennedy Duncan.
   (A. S. Barnes & Co., New York.)
Sound. Professor Tyndall.
   (Longmans, Green & Co., London.)
Mind and Body. Alexander Bain, LL.D.
   (D. Appleton & Co., New York.)

The Brain and Spinal Cord. Sir Victor Horsley.
   (Charles Griffin & Co., London.)
The Nervous System. Lewellys F. Barker, M.B.
   (D. Appleton & Co., New York.)
Anatomy of the Central Nervous System. Dr. Heinrich Obersteiner.
   (Charles Griffin & Co., London.)
Occult Chemistry. Annie Besant.
   (*The Theosophist,* beginning January, 1908.)

Printed in the United States
34370LVS00005B/12